MW00981710

Back from Obesity
My 252-pound Weight-loss Journey

Jan Bono

Sandridge Publications
Long Beach, Washington

First Printing, Fall, 2014

Printed in the United States of America
Gorham Printing, Centralia, WA 98531

Sandridge Publications
P.O. Box 278
Long Beach, WA   98631

http://www.JanBonoBooks.com

ISBN: 978-0-9906148-0-7

DEDICATED

to all who suffer from compulsive eating disorders,
with the hope that my story will both
inspire and encourage you,
and a gentle reminder that you are not alone.

ACKNOWLEDGEMENTS

Gratefully, and with much love, I'd like to thank all the
various "Eskimos," cheerleaders, partners in recovery,
support group friends, spiritual gurus, and glorious guides
of all types who have tirelessly aided and assisted me in my
continued program of weight-loss recovery.
Here are just a few, in the order of their appearance:

Jill, Estelle, Celia, New York David, Maggie, Miki, Steve,
my Law of Attraction guru, Michael Losier,
whom I've had the pleasure of meeting twice,
and Dr. Mehmet Oz, whom I expect to meet someday soon!

OTHER BOOKS BY JAN BONO

Collections of humorous personal experience:

Through My Looking Glass
The View from the Beach

Through My Looking Glass, Volume II

It's Christmas!
Forty-three stories and three one-act plays

Just Joshin'
A Year in the Life of a Not-so-ordinary
4th Grade Kid

Fiction:

Romance 101:
Forty-two Sweet, Light, Delicious,
G-Rated Short Stories

Poetry Chapbooks:

Bar Talk
Chasing Rainbows

A number of Jan's books are now available as eBooks on Smashwords.com. Find them at:

http://www.smashwords.com/profile/view/JanBonoBooks

INTRODUCTION

In 1998, I weighed 396 pounds.

That is not a typo. In 1998, I stood 5'6" tall and weighed Three Hundred Ninety-Six pounds. I'd tipped the scale, when I could find one that went that high, at over 370 for nearly a decade. A 60-inch measuring tape was not long enough to record my bust, waist, or hip measurements. I'd lost all hope of ever being a healthy weight or size again, and frequently wondered why I didn't just kill myself and get my whole miserable life over with.

But by some miracle I still can't explain, and quite a few supportive people who magically appeared in my life just when I needed them most, I found my bootstraps, and started the arduous process of reclaiming a body I wasn't ashamed of, along with my missing self-esteem.

Four years later, in 2002, I weighed a comfortable 168, without having used diet pills, any type of bypass surgery, and no extreme dieting or exercise to get there.

I maintained that weight for three years, and then the unthinkable happened: I relapsed. The reasons were many—relationships, retirement, resting on my laurels—but a compulsive overeater doesn't *need* a reason to overeat. The bottom line is that for those of us who have struggled with our weight our entire lives, a "reason" is just another word for "excuse."

During the next eight years, from 2005 to 2013, I regained a full 100 pounds. My whole life, not to mention the manuscript I'd written (*but never published*) about my weight-loss journey during the time I'd been "at goal weight," made me feel like one big, fat, fraud.

On January 1st, 2013, I weighed 255 pounds. My orthopedic surgeon told me I was too great a risk for him to consider knee replacement, and the physical pain was often unbearable. The emotional pain, of having recently achieved, and then lost, my healthy weight was even worse.

God willing, I'd turn 60 in June, 2014, and I desperately wanted to face that milestone with a body that was as good as it could possibly be. "Here we go again," I told myself, and began doing what had worked in the past—and what I knew would work again—if I just kept doing it.

I re-enrolled the support of a few friends, ingested the weight-loss wisdom of Dr. Oz on television while I rode my recumbent bike, and kept track of everything I ate in a daily food journal.

As I write this, I am happily hovering inside my self-proclaimed acceptable "target range." The magic (*which really isn't magic at all once you decide to do what is necessary*) still worked, and my story, from my all-time high of 396, down to 168, back up to 255, then down to my present acceptable target weight range of 143-147, still screamed to be told.

So here it is. And it's my fervent hope that those who read this story—of twice running the gamut of utter hopelessness to joyful celebration—will be inspired and motivated to take their own lives in hand and become their healthiest size possible.

If I can do it, you can too.

Jan Bono
August, 2014

Back from Obesity
My 252-pound Weight-Loss Journey

INTRODUCTION 5

CHAPTER I: HOW I GOT SO FAT 11

    The 60s: Kid stuff
    The 70s: Late teens and early 20s
    The 80s: The "M" years
    The 90s: A decade of life above 350 pounds

CHAPTER II: THE TURNING POINT 43

    Three hundred ninety-six pounds of reality
    Counselor from Hell
    In lieu of a straitjacket: A 5-point plan
    Four of five's not all that bad
    Support groups are for losers and wimps
    Backhanded inspiration
    A commitmentphobe makes a major commitment
    Meeting #11
    Something to hold on to
    My New York cheerleader
    Eskimos
    A food plan for life
    Garnering more support
    Dream it; believe it

CHAPTER III: 50 POUNDS DOWN 86

Willpower vs. won't power
Broasted chicken and the banishing bra
Maggie and Miki and Me
Giving thanks for broccoli and other green things
Singing the car buying blues
Finding the willingness to be me
'Tis the season to gobble down the goodies
Happy New Year 2000
The telltale rocks
In glorious black and white

CHAPTER IV: 100 POUNDS DOWN 117

Crosses to bear
What does "under 300" feel like?
Flying Solo: The view from the back of the plane
Sin City
Facing down the Department of Drivers' Licensing
No greater gift
What price, commercial recovery centers?
Do-it-yourself retreat
Maggie and Miki revisited
Heigh-ho Silver, away!
A metaphorical fish tale
Going for a test drive

CHAPTER V: 150 POUNDS DOWN............... 150

Fatteningly ever after
Where others had just begun
Fashion sense
Aborted Bridge Walk

Happy first anniversary
Dear John
Consolation prize
Catering by Costco
All I want for Christmas
Jim who?
Dining out
February madness
Every excuse for a binge
Some pain, but no weight gain

CHAPTER VI: 200 POUNDS DOWN: "Oh my God!
   The first digit is a one!" 179

Scaling down
Shape-shifting
The great bra-buying ordeal
Birthday burn center blues
The dating game
Sound the retreat!
Tummy tuck information overload
That's what friends are for
Gratitude, gratitude, gratitude
Incremental friends
Willing to go to any lengths
Las Vegas land mines

CHAPTER VII: FIRST DOWN & GOAL TO GO 213

Super-sized garage sale
The last 10 to 30 pounds are the hardest
Maggie and Miki yet again
9/11—Sugar won't fix it
T minus 7 and counting

A long and arduous journey
10/10 of 01
Two arms! Two arms!
Licking the bottom of the brownie bowl
Kicking and screaming all the way to goal
"Cosmetic" surgery
No secrets in a small town
Living at Goal Weight

CHAPTER VIII: RELAPSE?! .... .249
     Are You Freakin' Kidding Me?

The Elephant Man and me
One big, fat, fraud
Once more, with enthusiasm
The Law of Attraction
Pedaling my ass off
In the land of Oz
My all-time favorite fruit
Staying the course—against all odds
But the goal line had moved!
One day at a time

EPILOGUE: So What's the Plan? 270

ABOUT THE AUTHOR 272

CHAPTER I: HOW I GOT SO FAT

The 60s: Kid Stuff

"A chubby baby is a healthy baby." That was the conventional wisdom in the 1950s, and I was born in 1954, right smack-dab in the middle of the "Boomers." By the time I entered kindergarten, I might have been a little hefty for my age, but nobody thought it was anything serious.

There were four children in the family; I was, and still am, the eldest. When the third child was born, we moved from the "Lake City" area of north Seattle to a split level home in Lynnwood, a few miles north. For several years, Dad commuted 20 miles each way to his job in downtown Seattle while we settled into a richer existence in the suburbs—"The land of opportunity."

The opportunity I most recall was the almost limitless availability of food. Everything revolved around it.

Throughout elementary school, when I got high marks on a test or a good report card, we celebrated with food. When I got blue ribbons for science fair projects or running races at field days, we splurged by going out to dinner, and it was often "prime rib all around." When I fell down and got a boo-boo, a cookie was right there to "comfort" me.

Comfort cookies. That's what they should have called them. Even now, saying their full name brings the mouth-watering smell rushing back: Nestle's Toll House Cookies. Packed full of sugar, flour, butter, shortening, chocolate chips and walnuts, Mom made sure there were always plastic Wonder Bread sacks in the freezer chock-full of homemade cookies to add to our school lunches.

Naturally, I learned to comfort myself by helping myself. All my inferiority feelings of not being good enough, smart enough, pretty enough, tall enough, thin enough, ad infinitum, played havoc with my pre-pubescent self-worth, but a cookie, or two, or three, or a dozen or more, could make it all better. At least temporarily—like until the sugar buzz wore off.

I didn't realize until much later that the cookies stolen from the freezer marked the beginning of my penchant for sneak eating. If no one saw when and what I ate, then no one could tell me I was eating too often and too much.

Soon Mom discovered the nearby Hostess day-old bakery, and the freezer suddenly contained not only cookies, but chocolate cream-filled cupcakes, Twinkies, Ho-Hos and Ding-Dongs. It was a virtual paradise for a compulsive eater. Nobody kept an inventory of these allegedly school lunch treats, so nobody ever missed how many I stole.

I ate the cupcakes frozen, holding them upside-down, gnawing on the bottom cake layer first, then the cream center, and finishing up by licking the rapidly-thawing fudge frosting off my fingertips.

At mealtimes, we were reminded of the good fortune of being born in America and told we had to sit at the kitchen table until we ate everything on our plates. "We will not waste food—not while children are starving in Africa."

Both my parents had been raised in small town poverty. My father's father was a Mississippi River fisherman; Mother's father was a southwest Washington dairy farmer.

At Dad's childhood dinner table, there might not be

enough baking powder biscuits to satisfy everyone who showed up to eat, so he and his brothers often hid a quantity of them between their knees under the table as the basket was first passed.

Mom frequently told us the creative ways Grandma prepared their meals based on either "spuds and applesauce" or "applesauce and spuds." Potatoes and apples were plentiful on the farm, but they sacrificed a chicken only on the occasion when company came for Sunday dinner. One chicken—just eight pieces if fried—so often Grandma made chicken and dumplings or chicken pot pie, always with plenty of potatoes.

I suppose with this in their respective backgrounds, it was always a matter of "waste not, want not." But even then, I failed to see how anyone eating more than they wanted in America could possibly help the starving children in Africa, and once I remember suggesting we send them our leftovers.

Not surprisingly, my parents didn't find my comment the least bit amusing, and I still had to sit at the table until my plate was empty.

J.P. Patches was the local television clown. I watched him before school almost every morning. He had an amazing "ICU2 TV" and could "tune in" to everyone viewing his show. He often wished us a Happy Birthday or told us to clean up our rooms or mentioned something unique happening in our lives. And he frequently read from his list of "Clean Plate Clubbers."

I wanted to be a "Patches' Pal." I wanted to hear my name read by J.P. on TV, and everyday I kept my plate licked clean just in case he might tune in to our house.

By the time I was 10 or 11, I had figured out the connection between my uncle working the audio on the J.P.

Patches Show and the frequency of our names being mentioned. It was about the same time I also figured out how to supply myself with non-stop candy bars.

"Hot lunch" at school was 32 cents. Every night Dad emptied his pocket change into a Mason "money jar" in the kitchen cupboard. When we bought hot lunch, Mom handed out a quarter, a nickel and two pennies to each of us. No one ever knew exactly how much change was in the jar on any given day—a fact I duly noted.

Candy bars were a nickel apiece at the grocery store, or six for 25 cents and a penny tax. The closest market was two blocks up and seven blocks over, an easy ride for a kid on a bicycle. And it was also easy to slip an occasional quarter and a penny out of the money jar without fear of it being missed. Sometimes I brazenly stole two quarters and two pennies.

I never shared any of my candy bars. Not when I had six, and not when I had twelve. I never took long to pick them out, and I never took long to eat them. They were always completely consumed long before I got back home. Milky Way, Three Musketeers, Snickers, Look, Big Hunk, and of course, M&M Peanuts. Sometimes I got one of each, and sometimes I opted for several bags of M&M Peanuts supplemented with Milky Ways.

On Saturdays we kids attended the matinee at the local movie theater. Because the candy prices inside were so expensive, we stopped at the store on the way and filled our pockets with every conceivable type of theater treat. Mike and Ike's, Good 'n' Plentys, Jujubes, Milk Duds, and chocolate covered raisins.

I don't remember many of the movies I saw, but I can still recall the feeling of happiness that spread through me when I had my pockets loaded with candy and was headed to the movies. Sometimes I ate 6, 12, or even 18 candy bars during the double feature. I discretely unwrapped them and stuffed the wrappers down into the seat cushions so my siblings wouldn't tattle about how many I'd had.

The weekends we didn't go to the movies, we went to see Grandpa. It was a full day and half-the-night round trip. Mom prepared for it by cooking all afternoon the previous day. Fried chicken, potato salad and applesauce cake were the staples. Throw in a few jumbo-sized bags of chips, a few cans of Hi-C orange drink and several bags of marshmallows and/or cookies, and we were all set.

I loved helping Mom make the potato salad. Dicing up potatoes and eggs and green onion and radish and mixing it all in with globs and globs of full-fat mayonnaise.

"Taste this," she'd say, feeding me a big spoonful. "What's it need?" And I always knew just what it needed. A little more mustard, a touch more salt, another shake or two of pepper. Then I'd have to taste it again. And again. If no one had been there to stop me, I would have eaten the entire enormous mixing bowl of potato salad and still been hungry for more. Craving the tangy taste of the salad dressing she used, I could never get enough.

On the return from Grandpa's, we four kids sprawled out in sleeping bags in the back of the station wagon. Mom and Dad often stopped for ice cream sundaes on the way home. If I pretended to be asleep, like the other kids actually were, I knew they would stop at the hamburger drive-in. Then I would suddenly "be awake" and get to finish Mom's butterscotch sundae. Sometimes they even got me one of my own.

Ice cream played a significant role in my formative years. Still does. But back then, there were always several half gallons of different flavors in the refrigerator freezer.

We never ate a regular "serving" in a petite dessert dish. When we had ice cream, we used the soup bowls and piled it on, along with plenty of sugary toppings.

Hershey's chocolate syrup could turn any flavor into a fudge-blasting treat, but as a kid I still preferred it topping rocky road or marshmallow ripple. As a pre-teen I discovered the combined qualities of chocolate syrup over peppermint candy and/or chocolate chip mint ice creams, and I often put them all together in one bowl.

"Popsicle Pete" drove his ice cream truck down our street several times a week. The bell alerting us to his presence made my mouth start to salivate like one of Pavlov's dogs.

For a dime, I could get a Fudgsicle or Sidewalk Sundae or a Nutty Buddy. Sometimes my mother reached in the money jar and gave us all dimes, and one for her, too. She often requested a Creamsicle, and we had to hurry back before hers melted instead of sitting right down on the curb and enjoying our treats.

But occasionally when we heard the ice cream truck coming Mom said "No," and that meant I'd have to find a way to get my fix without her approval. A dime was easy enough to come by, so all I had to do was scale the wooden six-foot high back fence and wait for the truck to go down the next street. But if I were going to go to all that trouble, then I wouldn't get just one cold confection. For a quarter I could get two, and change back, or for two quarters, five ice cream bars could be mine—*all mine!*

By the time I was 11, I got most of my clothes in the "Chubby girls" section at Sears. I wasn't too worried about it, since I was active and full of energy. I heard the grown-ups talking about "baby fat" and thought that's all the extra pounds amounted to. I figured when I became a teen, the weight would just drop away, so it was okay until then to eat as much as I wanted.

Being a responsible student, I always had my homework finished, so my sixth grade teacher "recommended me" to be one of the lunchroom helpers. Not only did this mean I got "free" hot lunch every day, but I also got to help finish up the leftovers, which often included the tea rolls we called "dough goddies." Naturally, I pocketed the 32¢ Mom had laid out on the counter to pay for my hot lunch.

When the family ate breakfast out, it was often when we were on the road for a weekend jaunt. Most often we ate at truck stop restaurants with truck stop portions. I always ordered what my folks ordered: Two eggs over easy, hash browns, sausage or bacon, and toast. The other kids, being younger, might settle for one or two pancakes, but not me.

When we got hamburgers and fries, my sister, nicknamed Skinny-Minnie, got a milkshake with her meal to "fatten her up" while the rest of us got sodas.

"It isn't fair!" I'd protest. "You like her better than you like me!" Frequently I'd either end up with my own shake to keep me quiet, or be allowed to finish hers if she didn't drink it all, which she rarely did.

Whole new opportunities for compulsive overeating opened up to me when I entered junior high. For starters, instead of being just a block from home, the school was a little over a mile away. I usually rode the bus, but if I left early enough, I could walk to school. Walking to school meant I had to go right by the Albertson's grocery store, and the aromas from their bakery permeated the surrounding air for blocks.

There were two things I loved about that bakery. The first was "Texas Donuts." Texas Donuts were a lot like regular glazed donuts, only they were the size of dinner plates. They were always warm, slightly gooey, and so fresh the dough softly compressed in my mouth with each bite. Best of all, two of them only cost a quarter!

The second best thing about this bakery was something called "Indian Bread." It was a big rounded loaf, like half a basketball. If you asked, they sliced it right there for you, while you watched, salivary glands already in high gear from the smell of fresh baked bread. On days when I walked to school with a few of my friends, we often bought a whole loaf, along with a stick of real butter, and sat right down on the curb in front of the store to enjoy it together. There were never any leftovers.

During 8th grade, McDonald's opened up a new restaurant right next to the school. Now I had a reason to dawdle after school and accidentally miss the bus so I'd have to walk home. An unlimited source of hamburgers, French fries and milkshakes was impossible to pass up. A burger back then was only 15¢, and I always had money for more than one.

Although a little heavier than most of my friends, it didn't stop me from joining in with all the extra-curricular junior high activities. With the extra energy burned by playing sports, I managed to keep my weight pretty constant. And participating in after school events meant there was usually enough time to run over to McDonald's for a quick snack before boarding the activity bus home.

I was still in junior high when I began babysitting for the neighbors. As soon as their kids fell asleep, I ransacked the refrigerator, the freezer, and all the kitchen cupboards, looking for something good to eat while I did my homework. A few of the people I sat for left me a snack, but I never stopped there. Never satisfied with a normal portion, I constantly foraged for more.

During the summer I earned money by picking strawberries. Six days a week I boarded the "berry bus," with a very sizeable lunch from home, and made the trek with other kids my age to the fields of the lower Skagit Valley. By the time we arrived, I had already eaten one of my sandwiches and some chips or cookies and usually considered eating my second sandwich before getting out there to work in the fields.

We kids weren't the only ones out there picking berries. Migrant workers, who lived in the shacks nearby, were already hard at it before we arrived each day, and worked hours more after we loaded the bus to leave. For the convenience of those workers, there was a small store set up where they could charge a few necessities against their coming paychecks.

Of course, the store also took cash. And they had, among the "necessities," a pretty good supply of candy. Soon I was gobbling up my entire lunch on the way to the fields and buying up to a dozen candy bars as soon as we got there to give me enough energy to sustain myself through the long, laborious day.

I suppose I could have filled up on fresh-off-the-vine strawberries, and later in the summer there were plump, juicy raspberries as well, but that just didn't appeal to me as much as chewy hunks of anything made primarily of sugar.

Yet I never considered I might have an eating disorder. My weight, miraculously, never went much above 150 and I had already reached my adult height of 5'6", so I never felt too out of place among my peers.

Had I looked then to my genetic composition, I might have figured out I was destined to be an overweight adult. My father, at 5'11", struggled his entire life, mostly unsuccessfully, to keep his weight below 240. His seven brothers and sisters were all more-or-less overweight. As far as I know, not one of them, male or female, spent much of their adult lives under 220 pounds. "Potential muscle," my father called it, patting his belly as he tried to suck it in.

But now and again Dad tried to trim down. He drank Metrocal canned shakes as replacement meals for a few days, but complained constantly of deprivation hunger pangs. I know for certain it did not improve his disposition. He always made a huge production out of his "sacrifice" to get in shape, but I don't ever recall any tangible or lasting evidence of his success.

Mother, who never had a bona fide "weight problem," fought to keep her average size constant by running up and down the stairs to the utility room with load after load of laundry, doing sit-ups, and keeping unavoidably active while she managed a household with four children all under the age of 13.

She bought boxes of "Ayds" chocolate chews, which, if several of the small candy-like caramels were taken with a large glass of hot water before meals, was supposed to curb your appetite. She wasn't oblivious to how chunky I'd become, and suggested I try them too.

They weren't too bad. For a few weeks I ate several every day before meals. It was like getting a little pre-meal chocolate fix and it didn't slow my eating down at all. Soon I began sneak eating them, too.

I had just turned 14 when puberty caught up with me. A certified young woman at last, I thought my baby fat would just drop right off.

Since my first period arrived in June, I figured I'd be able to pare down during the summer before entering high school. For some incredibly naive reason, I was eager and optimistic for the next leg of my school career. I had no inkling the food challenges of my life as a child in the 60s would continue to the 70s and quite a ways beyond.

The 70s: Late teens and early 20s

I entered my sophomore year of high school in September, 1969, at the age of 15. I was chunky, but not abnormally large. At least I didn't think so at the time. Hindsight, however, is 20/20, and I think I always knew in my heart it wasn't just my perpetual bad haircuts that kept me from fitting in with the popular kids.

While I might not have been cheerleader material, I had a strong junior high sports background and quickly aligned myself with the high school "lady jocks." Unfortunately, the school journalism junkies, if they bothered to report on girls' sports at all, frequently referred to all female athletes as Amazons, and constantly portrayed us in a most unflattering light.

One of the most painful experiences of my adolescence, and one that will unfortunately endure forever, is a photo taken of me throwing a shot put. I think it may have been the first time I'd ever thrown a shot put in my entire life. My style left a lot to be desired. My head is back, the veins on my neck stand out, and one can almost hear the grunt of extra effort as I hoisted that ball of heavy metal, attempting to score a few more points for the track team.

In an effort to garner top honors at each meet, all the track team members were asked to compete in both track and field events. I figured since I was pretty good at throwing a softball, I might be able to pick up the slack in the shot circle. I did, and I suffered for it at every turn. I don't think I ever lived down the reputation I got by throwing the shot my sophomore year.

Although I ran the 100-yard dash and the first leg of the 440-relay, and competed at District and State in both those events, it was that damned shot put picture they put in the yearbook—a black and white focal point for my shame.

In my junior year, I was determined to be known for my running and not my field events. I wanted the respect of my classmates. I especially wanted respect from the boys. I started training for the track season a full month before our official practice began.

Dipping into my babysitting money, I ordered new baby blue and white track shoes with half-inch steel spikes from the local sporting goods store. Since I was busy working out with several other ambitious girls every day after school, my father picked up my shoes for me.

When Dad handed over the shoebox, he also handed me a small sack from the drugstore. Inside was a red and yellow box of Dexatrim.

"The guy at the sporting goods store said you could take a half a second off your 100-yard dash time if you lost 5 or 10 pounds," he said. "He's never even see you, but when I told him what you weighed, he said he was sure you'd better your time by slimming down."

I was 5'6" and 145 pounds. I had just gotten into "spring training" after laying off sports for the winter (*we had no girls' basketball in those days*). In a couple weeks I would probably have dropped some of my weight anyway. And no doubt I would have improved my time through my concerted effort to get back into the best shape possible.

But I was so young, so naive, and so very anxious to please my father. I took the pills every day. I felt the caffeine buzz and the racing of my heart as I watched with delight while the pounds dropped and my speed improved. I got down to 130 pounds and did, indeed, shave a little over a half second from my time in the 100.

When our official turnouts began, I was running so well I qualified for the coveted anchor position on the 440-relay, but opted to blast out of the blocks and carry the baton on the first leg instead. It was a position I had held for several years and I enjoyed the adrenalin rush as the gun went off and my feet flew toward the first turn.

Our girls' track team won meet after meet that year. In solidarity, we wrote a protest letter to the school newspaper and got them to drop the "Amazon" routine. The sports editor, pulling a pun from the cinder tracks we ran upon, began calling us "Cinder-ellas." We considered it a victory.

Meanwhile, I worked most evenings and all day Saturdays at a Little League concession stand. Hot dogs were the meal of choice, and there were plenty of candy bars within easy reach at all times, so I partook of a little instant energy boost whenever I felt the urge.

It wasn't uncommon for me to consume many thousands of "extra" calories every day. After bingeing on quantities of unnecessary snacks, I used to go to the restroom and stick my finger way down my throat, but I was never able to "successfully" purge. I suppose I should be grateful I had no easily-triggered gag reflex, but I remember praying throughout my high school years for just six months of anorexia.

I kept popping Dexatrim daily, available without a prescription, so I could buy copious quantities without parental permission. I somehow convinced myself it didn't matter what I ate as long as I kept taking my diet pills. Often, when I wanted to eat more, I took far more than the recommended dosage.

Toward the end of track season we had a beach bonfire

and barbecue at the coach's house on the shore of Puget Sound. I could get a discount through the Little League concession stand, so I signed up to bring the hot dog buns. After the word "Buns,", I printed "Bono."

Henceforth, the coach and at least half the track team constantly referred to me as "Buns Bono." At first, I considered it a friendly nickname. Later I realized that many of them, particularly those who were naturally and/or uncommonly thin, were laughing at me behind my back. Laughing at me and my big butt.

I quit taking the diet pills during the summer. And even though I was fairly active with tennis and volleyball during fall term, I gained back all the weight I'd lost, plus some. Then came the holidays.

At the start of the track season my senior year, I weighed more than 160 pounds. I was frantic. I got back into the Dexatrim. I started eating nothing but "diet food" like cottage cheese and hard boiled eggs and grapefruit during the day, but at night, when no one was watching, I gobbled up candy bars, never suspecting I was addicted to the sugar rush. I just thought I needed a little "extra energy" to help me study.

Of course the weight wasn't disappearing, so I began exercising to excess. And I fasted. And one day I fainted at school. The school nurse wanted to call my parents. I think she thought I was pregnant or something. Somehow I convinced her I just had "low blood sugar" and she handed me a 1200-calorie diabetic diet.

Twelve hundred calories seemed like way too many to eat to lose any real weight, so I cut back to about 500 a day. Consequently, I was dizzy and light-headed and almost unable to do my studies. I had to force myself to eat more out of some sort of innate self-preservation. In hindsight, it was undoubtedly my Higher Power, coming to my rescue before I could totally self-destruct and do irreparable damage to my body through improper nutrition.

Again in my senior season, the track coach asked all the runners to pick up some field events to boost our team scores. The shot put was out. I had determined it was decidedly unfeminine, while the long jump looked oh-so-much-more graceful.

To make a long story a little shorter, early in March, while practicing the long jump, I landed incorrectly, tearing the cartilage in my left knee. I had surgery, followed by six weeks in a hip-to-toe plaster cast. My last high school spring sports' season was over before it began.

Suddenly, there was no point in dieting, or taking diet pills, or even in abstaining from every fattening "comfort food" I could get my hands on. My life had changed irrevocably. I was completely inconsolable—but I figured enough chocolate just might help.

There was no prom for me, as no one asked. And even if they had, it's unlikely I would have agreed to go. I would have blamed the cast on my leg, but the truth was no tent-dress on earth that would have made me feel the least bit attractive. By the time I graduated in June, I was up over 180 pounds, and couldn't have cared less.

Apathy over my size followed me to college in the fall and I gained what is often called "The Freshman Fifteen." I lived through yet another knee surgery, spent my first winter quarter on campus on crutches, and alternately feasted and fasted my way to some semblance of weight control. With all the wild swings of the numbers on the scale I could have been the poster girl for yo-yoing weight.

When I was "in love," I worked hard to keep my figure. When I was not in a relationship, I ate to numb the uncomfortable feelings that arose from thinking I'd been "dumped" and no guy would ever find me good enough to love for a lifetime. Little did I know I was establishing a life-long pattern.

I graduated from college at 220 pounds and interviewed for several dozen teaching jobs. Time after time I came in "runner-up" for the position, and each time I noted the person who got the job weighed a good 70 or 80 pounds less than me. I learned first-hand about sizeism. Weight discrimination was, and for the most part still is, alive and well in America.

Eventually I landed a teaching position, and in that first year I gained another 20 pounds. Stress eating, I think I called it; there was a lot of stress facing down fourth graders every day. Or so I rationalized.

My aunt clipped a "Dear Abby" column out of the newspaper and sent it to me. I'm sure she meant well. The writer told how upset she was at her niece's size. Said she didn't want her niece coming over and sitting on her furniture, as she was sure she'd break it. She said her niece had "such a pretty face" but was an embarrassment to the family. This allegedly well-meaning aunt asked "Dear Abby" how she could get her niece to lose some weight.

I can't begin to describe the pain I felt when I read this clipping. My aunt had written "this could be you" in the margin along with "you must do something about your weight." She had not included Abby's response.

Quite by chance, I saw the same column printed in the local newspaper. Abby had told the busybody aunt to mind her own business.

Sadly, my relationship with my aunt was never reconciled, and she died many years before I cared enough to feign any kind of control over my eating.

Meanwhile, my parents' marriage was deteriorating. If I didn't whole-heartedly agree with Dad, he accused me of being on Mom's side. If I went to see my father, my mother acted as if I had betrayed her. I felt like a frayed and frazzled rope in a no-win game of tug-of-war. The more I tried to remain neutral, the more they both vehemently insisted I had abandoned them.

So naturally, I turned to food, my old stand-by, to console me. And just as naturally, I constantly overate. I'm not blaming them, they didn't bend my elbow and force food into my mouth. I'm just saying it didn't take much for me to want to numb my feelings with food.

The following year I took a teaching position on the Long Beach peninsula. It's a beautiful area, but I was isolated and alone, often homesick. But because of the divorce, I no longer had a home to return to. My overeating escalated to new heights.

I decided to stick it out at the beach for a maximum of three years—just long enough for me to complete my master's degree. Then I could move "back to civilization."

But by then I had eaten my way up to 275 pounds. Although I doubted a woman of my size could find another teaching position elsewhere, I sent applications to every school district along the I-5 corridor. As I'd predicted, when the next school year began, I was still living "at the beach."

The 80s: The "M" Years

The first day of school, 1980, I stood out on the playground at recess monitoring the children as they romped about. The principal stood next to me, and we chatted amicably while we kept a watchful eye on our youthful charges.

"What would it take to get you to stay in this community?" he asked.

I shot him a look. "It's the first day of a new school year," I replied. "Who said I was leaving?"

He smiled. "It's hard for a single person in a small community. You've been here three years already. Three years is about the average for young, unmarried teachers. Especially female teachers."

"You're right." I sighed. "I've been thinking that if I don't connect with someone locally this year, then it is definitely time for me to move on."

"So what are you looking for?"

I laughed. "Anything but a smelly old commercial fisherman."

And the Divine Mind of the Universal Spirit heard my words and she laughed like crazy.

I met Mr. Ex just two months later. He was, of course, a smelly old commercial fisherman. I weighed 260 at the time, but was dieting with a vengeance. I knew I'd have to lose weight to be considered a viable candidate during teacher interviews the following spring.

But my weight didn't seem to faze this fellow—maybe that was the big attraction I had to him—here was a man who said my size didn't matter, and he seemed to mean it.

We were married the following November. I had starved myself to a respectable 168 by time we said, "I do." In hindsight, that was the dumbest thing I'd ever said.

Within just a few days of tying the knot, I discovered a few horse flies in the ointment of blessed matrimony. I had a steady income. I had medical and dental benefits. I had a savings account. He, I suddenly discovered, had neglected to pay three years back taxes, now plus penalties and interest, was in arrears with his child support, and had a string of debts and bills past due up and down the coast of two states. All this I found out a little too late.

Yet I had made a commitment—a covenant with God. "Till death do us part," I had said when we made our vows. There was no turning back now. It's only money, I told myself with a shrug. But deep down, I knew I was lying through my teeth.

My inability to adapt to such an unequal partnership pushed me hard back into my food addiction. By August, 1982, I was hanging onto 178 pounds by the skinlessness of my chicken breast. The last week of that month, a couple significant things happened: My grandfather passed away, and I attended my 10-year class reunion.

The reunion fell between grandfather's passing and his funeral. I was in no frame of mind to go, but I went anyway. The first former classmate I ran into looked me up and down with his once-familiar elevator eyes and said drolly, "I see you finally let yourself go."

That was all it took— just one cruel comment. In my pain and my shame, right there at the reunion dinner I began to eat and eat and eat. As always, I wanted to numb the sense of disillusionment and disappointment. I wanted to stuff down all those uncomfortable feelings of inadequacy and frustration and powerlessness. I wanted to fill the void inside with something—preferably a fattening something—to comfort me.

Gramps, my unsung hero and role model for living an autonomous and independent life, was gone. Gramps had also been my inspiration to enter the teaching field. His death left a large gap in the roots of my family tree, the only grandparent I had ever known.

The chasm of intellectual differences between my spouse and me seemed to widen with each passing day. I had somehow managed to marry a man whose own lack of education exacerbated his feelings of inadequacy and encouraged his propensity to bully. All too soon, I became the made-to-order target of his frustration. And his rage.

For a half dozen years, while walking on matrimonial eggshells in an attempt to avoid conflict and confrontation, I binged and starved, yo-yoing up and down the scale like a drunken piano player.

My ex seemed to prefer me fat. When I managed to lose a few pounds, he'd bring home a half-gallon of ice cream or ask me to bake him a pie. Just because I was dieting, he'd whine, didn't mean he had to give up his own goodies.

I should have recognized the pattern of spousal sabotage. My father had responded to my mother's efforts to keep her figure slim and trim in much the same way, with a constant supply of butter brickle ice cream and M&M peanuts.

Often, on payday or any other excuse, my ex suggested we eat dinner out, because, he told me, I'd worked hard, and I deserved it. And dinner out always meant I'd eat a little more, have a few more richer and more fat-laden foods than I would have had at home, and indulge myself even further by sharing a dessert.

My gall bladder finally said "enough is enough" and I had to have it removed. While I was in the hospital, I called home, but was unable to reach my then-husband. The phone rang and rang but no one was home, and the answering machine, which we always left on, didn't pick up.

Later he said since I'd be sexually out of commission for awhile, he'd been "out getting some nookie" and hadn't wanted to deal with any guilt messages on the machine when he got home, so he'd turned it off. At the time, I assumed he was kidding.

The gall bladder surgery was in June. I spent the whole summer recuperating; the refrigerator was my solace and constant companion.

I was tipping the scale dangerously close to 300 pounds when my ex suddenly announced I was "sexually unattractive" and refused to have anything at all to do with me. I began starving myself again. A part of me thought it was all my fault he was turning away in disgust, and I didn't blame him. Another part of me got angry. "As soon as I can get this ring off," I vowed, "he's history."

One early Sunday morning in August, 1988, I was sitting at the kitchen table writing a poem. It was an idyllic morning—I had a cup of tea, I'd watched two deer eating buttercups out on the lawn, and all seemed somehow right with the world.

My ex broke into my reverie when he stomped out of the bedroom and demanded I come back to bed. "You know I can't sleep right when you're not there."

I slid the piece of paper I'd been writing on across the table toward him. "I've been working on a poem," I said. "I think it's pretty good. Want to read it?"

I will never forget what he did and said next. The memory scarred as deeply into my brain as if he had used a branding iron. He laid his hand flat on top of the paper and balled his fingers into a clenched fist, crumpling the paper up beneath his hand as he did so. Then he turned and tossed my poem into the wood box next to the fireplace.

"When it's published and in a book, then I'll read it," he said. "Until then, it's just junk. Now come back to bed."

I stared at him, pain and anger flaring through me. I opened my mouth and closed it again several times. I couldn't breathe and my ears started ringing. I wanted to slap him across the face, but I didn't want to give him justification for hitting me back.

Tears welled up and I fought them, unwilling to give him the satisfaction of seeing me cry. I was 210 pounds. In a blind rage I tugged and pulled and strained with all my might and my wedding band finally let go of my finger. I laid it on the table in front of me, glared at him with total distain, and announced in an uncannily calm voice, "I want a divorce."

"A divorce?! Over one lousy poem?" he asked incredulously. Actually, I think he used the F-word instead of lousy, but the point was made.

"No," I replied. "I've wanted a divorce for a long time, but I will always remember this moment as the straw that broke the camel's back." I could feel the veins sticking out on my neck. "I'm very serious. I want a divorce. I will see an attorney in the morning, and you better start looking for another place to live."

His eyes narrowed and his whole face turned dark. I thought he might hit me—it wouldn't have been the first time—but he just turned on his heel and stomped back to bed, certain I was bluffing.

But I wasn't bluffing, and I promptly filed the necessary paperwork. Three months later, I was a free woman, but I soon discovered the "real world" had changed in my decade of absence.

Our divorce became final in December, 1988, and for the next six months I spent more time in bars than I did at home. I wanted to be with people, I rationalized, and there was no one at home to talk to. It surely couldn't hurt to stop for a couple drinks on the way home. But one drink always led to another, and often I was still there when the doors closed at 2 a.m., despite having to work the next day.

By the grace of God I was never stopped by the police on the way home. By the grace of God I was never in an accident. I thanked God each morning when I opened the garage door and saw my car parked inside. And I wondered, because I truly couldn't remember, if I had driven it home myself, or if someone had dropped me off.

For a full six months, I stopped at the bar nearly every night after work, and was uncontrollably drawn to them on weekends as well. Sometimes I'd walk in and just lay my left arm, wrist side up, on the bar and instruct the bartender to "skip the middle man and just inject the booze."

I think I was afraid if I didn't stop by the bar every day I'd miss something—some juicy bit of gossip, perhaps. Or maybe I was afraid it was me who wouldn't be missed, and I'd be all-too-quickly forgotten.

The residual pain from my divorce was almost unbearable. Alcohol, I discovered, numbed the pain much faster and more effectively than overeating. Yet more often than not, I left the bar and went next door for a sizzling patty melt buried beneath an enormous pile of French fries before heading for home. Loading up on as much grease and fat as I could get my hands on at midnight or later became my standard routine. The weight started piling back on in leaps and bounds.

It was an agonizing attempt at a very slow suicide.

More and more the unresolved issues of my marriage surfaced. I sought out a counselor, who held my hand as I struggled with how blind I had been, how much I had tolerated, and all the spousal use and abuse.

Yet worst of all was the feeling it was me, and not the marriage, that had failed. Standing at the altar, I had made a covenant with God when I spoke the words, "Till death do us part," and I had broken that covenant. I vacillated between thinking I hadn't tried hard enough to make it work, to wondering why I had waited so long to get out and away from a horribly unconscionable situation.

I sought out my minister, who assured me God had not wanted me to live a life controlled by fear and/or abuse. He assured me God had forgiven me many times over for my decision to divorce. But I could not, or would not, believe him. Even with the minister's help, and the help of my counselor, the disparity in my own mind wouldn't resolve.

I fantasized about taking my life on an almost daily basis. I picked out a cement bridge abutment 30 miles from home and practiced driving my car at excessive speeds toward it again and again on weekends. At 80, 85, 90 miles per hour I drove toward the bridge. For some reason, I'd arbitrarily decided I'd have to be going at least 100 miles an hour and not be wearing my seatbelt to insure instant death. I couldn't take a chance of having to live a long and emotionally painful life with any type of paralysis.

I considered what would happen if I missed hitting the abutment head on. I couldn't risk making a 10 mph mistake. And since I never pressed my car to go a full 100 mph, I never managed to turn the steering wheel enough to follow through with my plan. At the time, I called myself a big, fat, chicken, but now I see it was actually my Higher Power interceding on my behalf.

My weight, however, continued to skyrocket. I ate and ate and ate, stuffing down every uncomfortable feeling threatening my sanity. It was a virtual Catch 22. I was so fat, I wanted to die, so I ate even more and got even fatter.

My fat became a living chastity belt. I never wanted to be hurt by any man ever again, and I rationalized if I was fat enough, no man would want to come near me. I isolated myself with my food and sat out the rest of the 80s hiding in my house, compulsively eating behind drawn drapes, immersed in self-loathing.

As the decade closed, I started referring to it as the "M" years—Married—and I swore to never make the mistake of getting married ever again. I sought to shuck off the shame I'd felt for the crimes committed against me. I clung to the belief that with the 80s, and my marriage, behind me, the 90s gave me a fresh chance to start anew.

The 90s: A decade of life above 300 pounds

Obesity made the headlines time and again during the 1990s. First the scientific community declared it a genetic predisposition, giving angry overweight individuals one more thing to blame on their parents. Then the American Medical Association officially proclaimed obesity a disease. The Surgeon General concurred, and the Supreme Court said it was a bona fide disability covered by the Americans with Disabilities Act.

Insurance companies revolted, making cold-hearted "exceptions" to their coverage of those considered by the arbitrary weight standards to be "morbidly obese."

My minister stood in the pulpit one fine spring day and proclaimed obesity a sin—right along with drug abuse and alcoholism. He supported his position with Biblical references to the body being a temple, and I suppose it sounded all well and good and logical to the few of those sitting in the pews who did not suffer from any of the aforementioned maladies.

Compulsive eating is indeed a disease, and most probably occurs due to a genetic and/or chemical disorder, but I refused to feel one more shred of guilt or shame over being fat. My face burning with embarrassment, sure everyone in the congregation stared in my direction with either pity or disgust, I left the church immediately after the service, not staying for the usual fellowship afterwards.

I did not return to church the next week, or the next, or even during the next few years. If I couldn't feel unconditionally accepted within the sanctuary of my own church, where could I feel "safe?" I was a woman without a country—or at least without a temple of worship.

Full of indignant self-righteousness, I concluded I had suffered enough. I certainly didn't need to be treated this way. Let he or she who is perfect cast the first stone! Incensed, I felt singled out—metaphorically nailed to the cross for a modern-day persecution. Fat people were still "fair game."

Of course my reasoning was a tad bit faulty, but too far into my disease to understand that, I took it all quite personally. It was easy to see who was the fattest person in the congregation.

So I turned my back on the only avenue of spirituality I had ever known—organized religion—and sunk lower and lower into the major food groups of chocolate, fat, sugar and caffeine. If the food in front of me was loaded with empty calories, I shoved it in my mouth in ever-increasing quantities. An abhorrent form of self-medication, and I became powerless to stop doing it.

The nineties were my true decade of darkness. I began avoiding leaving the house except to go to work and gather more food. In the grocery store checkout lines, I found myself lying to the checker about needing "all this food" because I was having a big get-together over the weekend. Then I'd leave the store and drive to the next market and load up yet another overflowing shopping cart. I ate copious amounts of anything and everything, most of it behind closed curtains, all alone.

I continued to fantasize about having anorexia for just six good months and about what I would do if I awoke from a coma "suddenly thin." This daydream happened often while devouring a half-gallon of ice cream in a single sitting after the couple barely-baked frozen pizzas I'd polished off an hour before.

Every so often I made a half-hearted attempt at "dieting." I read hundreds of magazine articles on the subject and tried nearly as many different "miracle cures." The cottage cheese and grapefruit and hard-boiled egg "diet" so popular in the 60s was only the tip of the iceberg.

I tried no carbohydrates, just carbohydrates, high protein, low protein, Hilton Head and Atkins. I tried eating nothing but cabbage soup for several weeks. I drank buckets of water before every meal. I tried eating only one meal a day. Then self-diagnosing hypoglycemia, I began eating six meals a day, and not a single one of them qualified as "small."

I experimented with various diet aids and pills. The back pages of the magazines I read were full of "Amazing Weight Loss" tales. From fat blockers promising the calories in the food I ate would pass through my intestines unabsorbed, to a plastic wrap that guaranteed I would shrink a full size by morning, I was lured by the promise of someday looking like a "normal" person.

But I wasn't normal, and I needed to come to terms with the idea I would never be normal. If losing weight was truly simple, and keeping it off ultimately easy, there would be no overweight epidemic. No one chooses to be a compulsive eater; we are simply, and sadly, born that way.

And yet I continued to look for the "quick fix." I researched the surgical options: Stomach staples, gastric bypasses, balloons and sponges inserted into the body to give a false feeling of "fullness."

Surgery, however, is not high on my list of fun things to do. I passed up those extreme measures because no one I had ever met who had undergone a single one of these procedures was glad they had gone that route. There were just too many complications.

For some unexplainable reason, Xenical, Merida, Phen-fen, and all the rest of the miracle drugs of the decade also failed to hook me with their attractive promises of rapid weight loss. My tango with Dexatrim in the early 70s, quite possibly at the root of my adult eating disorder, had convinced me pills often did more harm than good. Or perhaps the list of possible side effects for many of these fat-blocker drugs dissuaded me. Bolting from my classroom for the bathroom whenever the "gaseous discharges," a.k.a. diarrhea, took control of my internal workings was not acceptable.

One day I read a hypnotherapist's ad in the local newspaper. Grasping at yet another panacea, I committed to four sessions with the hypnotist. If it worked for smokers, and those afraid to fly, why not with food addictions and portion control?

Four weeks later the hypnotherapist had stirred up many unresolved issues from my childhood, but I had lost no weight. I discontinued my appointments, but made a lifelong compassionate friend.

Three Januarys in a row I signed up with TOPS (*Take Off Pounds Sensibly*). My first meeting I weighed in at 372. And while the program "worked" for a few months, and I dropped a little over 50 pounds, the next January I found myself back at exactly the same weight. The very same starting weight! Nonetheless, I signed up again. And another year passed with almost identical results.

The following January I enrolled in the 12-week "Eating Slim" program sponsored in part by the Oregon Dairy Council. Each week I drove to Columbia Memorial Hospital in Astoria and weighed in and listened attentively to the instructor, a little waif of a nutritionist. I followed the plan, marked my food groups and portions on their prescribed charts, and lost some weight. But when the class was over, I regained everything I'd lost in half the time.

I tried exercising. Nothing too serious or strenuous, just walking a short distance along the road near my home. Teen-agers out cruising aimed their cars at me and yelled for me to "get that fat butt off the roadway." I waddled home in shame, laughed at for attempting to exercise and laughed at for being fat. I couldn't win. I considered a long walk on the beach, heading due west.

In the 90s it became "politically incorrect" to make jokes about Polacks, blondes, gays, stupid Senators, and a host of other "minority" groups. But so-called comedians, such as Jay Leno, never missed an opportunity to mock and ridicule celebrities like Elizabeth Taylor, whose weight issues were often plastered all over newsstand magazine covers. Fat people, said Leno, "make such an easy target."

As my weight continued upward, my wardrobe shrank. Lane Bryant and Roaman's catalogs were my only option. Time after time I ordered clothing not because I liked the outfit, but because it came in a size big enough. Size 60 or 6X was as high as the numbers went, so that's what I purchased. The majority of the time I had to send back clothes that wouldn't go around me, paying the cost of shipping and handling in both directions, but ending up with nothing new to disguise my body.

All my pants were elastic-waist polyester pull-ons. Black, dark blue, and brown. Almost every blouse I owned was the same shapeless "A-frame" style, long-sleeved to hide the rolls of arm flab between my elbow and armpit and at least 30 inches long in hopes of camouflaging the enormous overhang of my stomach.

When I managed to find something reasonably attractive that covered me, my coworkers were quick to notice my new clothes. Unable to take any kind of a compliment, I poked fun at myself, joking that I bought it at "Omar's Tent and Awning."

Sometime during the early 90s I stopped taking baths. I loved bubble baths after a hard day at work, but I was forced to give them up. I couldn't bend far enough to gently lower myself into the tub without falling, and I feared that I would not be able to get my legs pulled in under me to stagger to my feet and step out unassisted. I could still cram my hips into the tub, but the size of them sealed off the water so effectively that none of the liquid flowed behind me once I was wedged in.

And even with all this humiliation, with all my lack of self-esteem, with all the fingers of society pointing at me and telling me I was a walking eyesore to the rest of humanity, I still knew somewhere deep inside me, I was a very good person, and certainly worthy of a loving romantic relationship.

Unfortunately, I was probably the only one who unequivocally knew this. But forever the slightly-delusional optimist, I answered personal ads, and placed a few myself. The storyline was always the same. "You're how big?" "Thanks, but no thanks."

Once while driving on I-5, a trucker hailed me on the

CB radio. He said he "had a little time," and would I like to stop for coffee? But when I got out of my car, he took one look at me and got back into his truck, saying, "I haven't got *that much* time."

I grew even more bitter and resentful. How could these men not see what a wonderful person I was? What a bunch of stupid jerks! How narrow-minded! What was the matter with them?! So of course, I ate, numbing the pain of rejection after rejection.

I tried turning to my female friends for comfort. I asked them to "set me up" on blind dates. None of them ever did. They claimed they didn't know anyone "as intelligent" as me, and said they knew only a "smart man" would do.

In reality, my size made me the worst kind of social outcast. Whereas an alcoholic, drug addict, spouse or child abuser can hide his or her true disposition for a period of time, obesity is right out there, the first thing anyone ever sees. Most of the time, the *only* thing anyone saw.

To satisfy my longing for intimate connections, I began reading romance novels. But none of them ever had a female protagonist larger than a size 6. Their definition of "gorgeous" always contained the words thin, trim, petite, attractive, svelte, slim or slender. In defiance, I wrote a short story for Woman's World Magazine in which the main character was a "larger," yet quite active and definitely fit woman. The editor rejected my story, stating that it "doesn't meet our readership needs."

I broke all the rules of freelance writing and wrote the editor back, reminding her that this was the same "readership" who bought the magazine each week with women and their weight loss stories dominating every cover. I asked her if she thought larger women had the right to feel sexy and romantic. The editor did not respond.

(Meanwhile, the same magazine carried articles citing the number of calories you can burn by chewing gum or clicking your computer mouse!)

In near desperation, I began accessing online chat rooms, exploring the crazy world of cyber relationships. "What do you look like?" the men asked me. "You tell me," I replied, "and I'll be your fantasy girl." When pressed further, I described myself as having "an hourglass figure with plenty of time to spare for the right guy." For years, the closest I came to having a "date" was deep within the make-believe world of cyberspace.

By the middle of 1999, my life had deteriorated to not much more than go to work, come home, get online for hours, and eat and eat and eat. And my now dangerously close to 400-pound life was no life at all.

CHAPTER II: THE TURNING POINT

Three hundred ninety-six pounds of reality

I wasn't a very nice person. I hadn't been a very nice person for quite a long time. I should have changed my name to B.A.R.B.—Bitter, Angry, Resentful Bitch. I blamed everything from "inherited fat genes" to an uncaring and punishing God for my innumerable problems, obesity being at the very top of the incredibly lengthy list.

No wonder I didn't have a lot of friends—I didn't even like me, so how could anyone else? Deep inside, I had known for over a decade something would have to change, and I even suspected that the change had to come from within me. But for years I honestly didn't know where, or how, to begin. I lived with constant hopelessness, and it would have to be an act of God, in the form of a miracle, to move me to take the first small step.

It was my bed that finally did it. If there were one single event, one moment in time that finally got me to acknowledge my morbid obesity and rapidly diminishing health, I'd have to point to the day my 18-year-old waterbed mattress gave up its last seam.

Why God used the demise of my waterbed to get my attention is beyond me, but He did, and I'm forever grateful. The way I figure it, the fact I'm here to tell this story today is evidence of a power greater than myself—a power guiding me back from imminent premature death to a full, rewarding life.

For the purpose of simplicity, I'll call that power "God," but you can call it by any name that makes you comfortable: Higher Power, Energy Source, Divine Spirit, Universal Mind, Collective Consciousness—it doesn't matter. The point is, something "out there," or maybe something living inside me all the time but heretofore unacknowledged, helped turn my life around. Praise be to whatever force, by whatever name you choose.

My story of weight-loss recovery begins on a sunny March morning in 1999, when I awoke to a primal sensation of rebirthing. Even before I opened my eyes, I realized the waterbed bladder had finally burst. As I sloshed wearily over the padded side railing, I knew in my heart it was time to grow up and get a "real" bed.

Unfortunately, trying to sleep in a "real" bed had immediate drawbacks. There was no way I could get my body comfortable enough to sleep.

I tossed and turned and cursed the apparent inability of mattress makers to create a satisfactory product. First one hip hurt, I'd roll over, and then the other hip almost immediately began aching. I couldn't rest on my back at all. After 18 years in a warm and coddling sleep environment, I was suddenly forced to lie on a relatively hard, unyielding, and extremely unforgiving mattress.

A couple months passed. I wasn't able to lie in one position for more than 20 or 30 minutes without waking up in pain—the kind of pain that often necessitated getting out of bed and walking around for a little while. I dreaded the coming of each night, apprehensive about getting enough sleep to make it through the next day. I began taking two, or maybe three Tylenol P.M. at bedtime, but even they gave me very little relief.

Somehow I finished my 23rd year of teaching and hoped during the summer, without the stress of having to get up early for school, I'd be able to relax and get caught up on my rest.

But by the end of June I doubted I'd ever get a full hour's sleep again. I awoke with a start every few minutes, gasping for breath. I'd always been a stomach sleeper, and now I damned the mattress for pressing so hard against my rib cage that breathing was difficult, if not impossible. Lying on my stomach, unable to lift my own bulk with enough air to fill my lungs, there was the very real danger of suffocating. Most nights I ended up sleeping in the recliner in the living room.

I self-diagnosed sleep apnea, and knew my obesity had a great deal to do with it. Desperately needing sleep, I reluctantly made an appointment with my Physician's Assistant for a complete physical—but all I wanted was for her to write me a prescription for a decent sleep aid.

My Physician's Assistant ran all the usual tests. Oddly enough, everything seemed to be perfectly normal. Blood pressure, blood sugars, iron, thyroid, cholesterol—all were within the acceptable range. But the elephant sitting on the examination table couldn't be ignored forever.

"How much do you think you weigh?" asked my P.A. She already knew her nurse had not been able to record my true mass using their limited office scale.

This hadn't surprised me. No doctors' scales in my county or the next had the capacity to go above 350 pounds. I'd checked clinics and hospitals everywhere, and eventually found a small local meeting of TOPS (*Take Off Pounds Sensibly*) where they had a scale that recorded weight as high as mine.

"I'm 396," I told my P.A. without flinching. "Dressed, but without shoes."

My P.A. didn't flinch either. Nor did she begin to lecture. She simply looked at me, looked again at my chart, inhaled deeply, slowly exhaled, then softly said, "I'd like to send you to a counselor."

A counselor? I had come in for a physical exam because I couldn't sleep. All I needed were some good sleeping pills; I certainly didn't need a shrink. Lots of women were "supersized." *Somebody* had to be the fattest so everyone else could feel good about themselves—

I took my own deep breath and counted to 10 before responding, and when I did, I think the soft tone of my voice surprised us both. "Why do you think I should see a counselor?"

"I think you have PTSD," she continued quietly.

"*PTSD?*" I couldn't believe what I'd just heard. "*Post Traumatic Stress Disorder?*" I asked incredulously. "Are you kidding me? I've never even *been* to Vietnam!" I tried to make light of her diagnosis by laughing it off.

"Haven't you just emerged from a war zone?" she asked, referring to my year with a particularly difficult group of junior high students. "Wasn't being at work like being in a constant battlefield?"

I had to agree. But the school year was behind me now— it was *over.* O-v-e-r. Why couldn't I just forget it, let it go, move on, and get some sleeping pills so I could sleep?

My P.A. tore a page off her prescription pad and handed me the paper. There was a phone number on it. "She's a very good counselor," she said. "I think you'll like her." She paused. "And I think she'll be able to help you."

I had just turned 45. I weighed a mere smidgen under 400 pounds. Often short of breath after very little exertion, I had frequent dizzy spells. My bladder leaked when I sneezed or coughed. Bending down to tie my own shoes was the only aerobic exercise I got. I wasn't able to sleep even half an hour without struggling for air. I went through all kinds of contortions in the bathroom each day in order to perform the most basic personal hygiene.

Since I considered myself a fairly intelligent human being, I knew it was time. Past time. When it hurts more to suffer than to change, perhaps it's time to change.

With barely two months before school resumed, I didn't think I had the stamina to face another class in my current condition.

I called the counselor and made an appointment.

Counselor from Hell

The counselor turned out to be a fiery redheaded woman in her early 50s with a penchant for southwestern Native American art. She wore a long suede skirt and cowboy boots. She spoke her mind, listened to few excuses, and took no prisoners.

Trained in EMDR *(Eye Movement Desensitization and Reprogramming),* she tried unlocking the traumas that had driven me to hide behind my size. She saw my weight as nothing more than a symptom—a deadly symptom of too much stress and too little perceived control over my own life. I was obviously self-medicating with food. I ate to cope with daily stresses; I ate to numb the constant internal pain; I ate because it gave me comfort. Or so I thought.

Even though it was slowly killing me, I didn't want to give up the food. I liked being able to eat whatever I wanted and as much as I wanted. My blood pressure and cholesterol were both fine, I reminded her. I was there because I couldn't get a good night's sleep. I told her to lay off nagging about the food thing. Eating was one of a very few activities that still gave me any kind of pleasure.

During our third session, the counselor suddenly wheeled her office chair over in front of the couch where I sat, grabbed the fabric of my blouse below my throat and yanked my head uncomfortably close to hers.

"*Do you want to die?!*" she screamed in my face.

I stared at her. I swallowed. Then I blinked. I blinked and she didn't. She held her ground, with her face just inches from mine, and patiently waited for me to answer her question.

I have no idea how long we sat there like that. It seemed like ages, but it was probably a little less than 30 seconds. My thoughts whirled and I felt a strong wave of nausea as I struggled for the words—or the will—to answer her honestly. Did I want to die? What kind of a question was that?

In an uncharacteristically small voice, I finally answered her. "Do I have a choice?"   She nodded, released her grip on my blouse, and backed off a few feet. "I want you to go to an inpatient program for 28 days."

"No way."

"Do you want to get better?"

"Yes."

"Are you willing to go to any lengths to get better?"

"I will not go to a treatment center. That's for alcoholics and drug addicts. I don't want the stigma. I'm a teacher in a small town. I can't possibly go to an inpatient program, even if I wanted to—which I don't."

"I see," she said, nodding again. "So you think it's better to die 'looking good' rather than risk being labeled a compulsive overeater?"

I had no answer for that.

"Don't you think the people in this community can take

one look at you and see something's very wrong?" She paused, tilted her head and asked, "You think you're fooling anybody?"

I still said nothing.

She waited.

We participated in another silent stare down for several more minutes. Again, I cracked first.

"What else can I do *besides* go to an inpatient treatment center?"

The counselor raised an eyebrow at me.

"Just tell me what to do. Give me a lesson plan; I can follow a lesson plan. I was *born* to follow a lesson plan. Damn it! Just tell me what to do!"

I'm sure she heard the desperation in my voice, and I'm sure she didn't believe I could do what was necessary 'on my own.' She considered her response for a few moments, then quietly said, "Okay, first we'll try it your way. Write this down."

I flipped open my ever-present stenographer's notepad and wrote as she dictated.

In lieu of a straitjacket: A 5-point plan

I didn't like what the counselor told me I'd have to do, but I knew I could never go to inpatient treatment. Never in a million years. What possible lasting good would it do me? What lasting good had it ever done anyone?

After 28 days you come back home to the same old, same old, and nothing has really changed. I'd seen numerous people return from alcohol treatment centers and dash straight to the nearest bar, eager to make up for a month of teetotaling.

How could I hope to return from a 28-day food addict's funny farm and maintain the momentum needed for the kind of weight-loss I ultimately faced. I could only imagine what all I'd eat when I got out, making up for a month of inconceivable food deprivation. Before it came to that, I resolved to give the counselor's suggestions my best effort.

The next morning, I dutifully reviewed my "to-do" list:

1) <u>Start taking vitamin supplements and antioxidants</u>. The focus was on vitamins A, C, E, selenium, calcium, glucosamine and chondroitin. With many arthritic problems in my knees, the last two suggestions were primarily for joint pain relief.

2) <u>Eat sensibly</u>. What in the world did *that* mean? Find a diet? *Another* diet? Count calories? Cut out sugar? Eliminate white flour? Carbohydrates? Caffeine? Here we go again, I thought, but "dieting" was something I knew a lot about. I'd been on and off diets since I was a teen-ager. I hated carrot and celery sticks with a passion. I'm not a slug, a snail, or a rabbit, and I refused to voluntarily spend the rest of my pitiful life eating like one!

3) <u>Get some exercise</u>. Getting out of bed, showering, and pulling on my clothes was nearly too much for me. The first day I decided to walk to the end of my driveway and back without stopping. I quickly discovered that wasn't possible, stopping twice during a less-than-100-yard stroll.

4) <u>Attend a support group</u>. No way. I'd tried too many already. All the people I met there were women who griped about how much they ate all week and then complained when the scale reinforced the truth behind their behavior. People who attended support meetings were just looking for the social aspects of going to a group. They were weak. Woosies. Wimps. A strong person could lose weight on his or her own. I, of course, was a strong person.

5) <u>Get a cat</u>. *Get a cat*? Are you kidding me? What in the world do I need a *cat* for? But my counselor had explained living as a single woman, I had no one to care for, no one who needed me, no one for whom I was responsible. She suggested if I had a cat, at least I would get my butt out of bed on weekends, because the cat would need feeding. Well, okay. Maybe. At least a cat wasn't as demanding as a dog.

The goal here was avoiding inpatient treatment. To avoid that, I would do almost anything. *Almost*.

Four of five's not all that bad

"Get your homework done?" asked my counselor the next week.

"I got a cat." I glowered at her.

"You got a cat?"

"Yes, as I just told you, I got a cat. Must you insist upon repeating everything I say?"

"What did you name your cat?"

"I named him Bubba."

"Bubba?"

"Yes, Bubba." I avoided making eye contact.

"I see." My counselor reviewed her notes. "What about the other things I told you to do?"

I sighed. "Well, I've started taking the vitamins and supplements."

"Good."

"And I walked a little."

"Goooood." She strung the word out until it sounded like it had several extra syllables.

"And I've been writing down what I'm actually eating

so I'll know the difference when I start eating healthier."

"Hhhmmmm." She waited for several seconds, but when I did not offer up anything more, she finally asked, "And what support group meeting did you attend?"

I sidestepped her question. "I went down to the Humane Society and sat in the cat room waiting for one of the cats to pick me. It took three days. I haven't had time to look into support groups yet, but hey, I got a good start on four of your five suggestions."

"*Suggestions?*" She raised an eyebrow, but said nothing more. She just looked at me, waiting. We sat in silence. The silence, as usual, grew uncomfortably long. Not only could this woman go for hours without blinking, but she was an absolute expert at sitting in silence. Finally, I could bear it no longer.

"Hey! I exclaimed defensively, "I got the damn cat! I didn't want a cat, but I got one. At least that's something! You got to give me some credit, here! I got an effing *CAT*, for crying out loud!

Support groups are for losers and wimps

No doubt about it, I had a crummy attitude. Over the years, I had attended a wide variety of diet groups, clubs, programs, weight-loss centers with their own food to purchase, and hospital-sponsored nutrition classes. Often, the only two things required were pay the admission fee and step on the scale each week to record your weight. I could save a great deal of money by just stepping on the scale at home.

The last thing I needed was failing publicly. Again. So support groups were definitely out. But according to my absolute shrew of a counselor, support group attendance was mandatory if I wanted to keep myself out of a treatment center. But what the hell did she know?

"Are you willing to go to any lengths?" she had asked me. I thought about that. A lot. Had I tried absolutely *everything*? Had I left no stone unturned in my desire to suddenly wake up thin one morning? What did I really have to lose? (*About 240 pounds, I told myself, and laughed aloud at my own morbid joke.*)

I found the phone number for the contact person of the group my counselor had recommended and clipped it out of the newspaper. I waved it in her face during my regular session the next week. "See? I'm getting closer," I said. "I'm making progress."

She said nothing. Blast that woman's poignant silences!

The day before my next counseling appointment I actually picked up the telephone. It took everything I had not to hang up when a live person answered my call. I was hoping for an answering machine, and had a practiced noncommittal message all ready. I hadn't yet decided if I'd leave my phone number—probably not.

The woman who answered my call had far too much peppy energy to be very much overweight. She cheerfully answered all my questions, then told me she looked forward to seeing me at the next meeting.

I wasn't too sure about any of this, and her sunshine and roses attitude didn't help at all. I didn't do chipper, and I didn't do perky, and I figured the woman had to be high on something to talk with me the way she did. Life was a bitch, and she couldn't convince me otherwise.

"Have you gone to a support group?" asked my counselor as soon as I sat down the following day.

"They only meet on Saturdays," I said smugly.

"And are you going to go to next Saturday's meeting?"

I sighed. I pointedly looked around the room at her collection of western art, avoiding her eyes. Finally, I sighed heavily and asked, "Is it absolutely necessary?"

"Yes," she replied in her no-nonsense manner, "it most certainly is."

"Ok. Fine. Whatever." I shrugged. "I'll go."

"You don't have to like it," she said. "But you must go."

So the following Saturday, promptly at 10:20 a.m., I sat in my car and watched as a dozen other women, of all assorted shapes and sizes, went inside the meeting room. There were women who looked height/weight proportionate, a few who looked downright thin, some who looked about my size, and everything in between. By my calculations, I wouldn't be the biggest, but I'd probably be the first runner-up.

Finally, at 10:29, I got out of my car and waddled toward the building. It was the longest walk I'd taken in years. Literally, as well as figuratively. There were four short stairs to navigate before I got to the door. At the foot of the steps I again considered turning around and leaving. My heart pounded, probably more from my exertion than actual fear, but I couldn't be sure. Short of breath, I leaned against the stair railing.

The screen door above me swung open and I was enthusiastically welcomed by the woman I had spoken with on the phone. There was no mistaking her vibrant attitude and voice, and her smile, which seemed to take up her whole face, was not only large, but seemingly genuine.

She held out her hand to help me mount the stairs; I hoisted myself up one painful step at a time. Once inside, she handed me a "Newcomer's Packet" stuffed with pamphlets and information about the group. I shoved it into my purse and scanned the room for a place to sit. I hesitated, sure none of the still-available chairs would hold my bulk. Intuitively understanding my dilemma, a few of the women already seated shifted places, clearing a space for me at the end of one couch.

As the meeting got underway, I took a good look at my surroundings. Candles. Lots and lots of candles. I felt like I was in some type of incense-filled cathedral. Or maybe a wake. The meeting began with a short prayer, which I had heard before but did not know by heart, and within the first three minutes I was absolutely certain I didn't belong here. I kept this insight to myself, and didn't say a word during the meeting. Not a single word. I had fulfilled my counselor's requirement—I had attended.

I listened with only half an ear, my eyes watching as the hands of the clock crept ever-so-slowly toward noon, impatient for my release from this horrific discomfort, which steadily grew as the meeting wore on. I didn't appreciate what I was hearing, and I didn't know what possible benefit I could get from listening to the sordid stories these women told, so I basically tuned them all out and focused on the flame of the candle nearest me.

But somehow a few things crept into my consciousness anyway, for I found myself nodding with understanding as one woman explained "the three-legged stool."

She said we were all compulsive overeaters. *(Well, duh!)* But to "recover" we had to get our emotional, spiritual, *and* physical programs in sync, and then work to keep them in harmony. Our "stools" could not balance on one or two legs; we needed all three supports in place.

I'm a very visual learner. My mind drifted back to when I was a kid, and the milk stool in my uncle's barn. I thought how funny it would have been to see him try balancing on one or two legs of the stool while he milked the cows. I smiled at the image.

But I'm not like these other people here, I told myself again. All I have to do is quit eating so much. They talk too much about God; I don't need all this God stuff. What does my "level of spiritual fitness," as they called it, have to do with losing weight? I understood the emotional piece. That was simple. I readily acknowledged how my emotional state determined how much, and what, I was eating.

I already *knew* I ate for every conceivable reason under the sun. I ate to celebrate, to mourn, and out of sheer boredom. I already *knew* I ate to "numb the pain" and shove down uncomfortable feelings. I already *knew* my overeating had more to do with "self-medicating" and poor coping skills than it did with hunger.

The physical leg of the program was all I had come for. Just tell me what to do to quickly lose this much weight. The quicker the better. I had only come to this meeting to get another diet and be done with it. Where was the diet? *Just show me the damn diet!*

"We are not a diet and calories club," the introduction to the meeting had explained. Right then and there I knew this program, this so-called support group, would never work for me. At the meeting's conclusion, I dodged most of the hugs and well-wishes for the week and bolted, as best as a woman of my girth could, for the door. No way would I be coming back. No way in hell.

I drove a few blocks, pulled into a grocery store parking lot, and suddenly found the energy to grab a cart and lumber rapidly down the center aisle, nearly running people over in my haste to get to the frozen food department.

At the meeting I had heard one woman say we could

either admit we were powerless over compulsive eating, or we could prove it. *Heck, I could prove it just fine*, I snickered to myself. I admitted I was powerless over Ben and Jerry's ice cream, and reached eagerly for my favorite flavor. Okay, make that flavors—I knew there was no way that just one pint was going to be enough. Not today.

I ate an entire pint of "Phish Food" ice cream on the ride home. Dark chocolate with little darker chocolate fish candies liberally sprinkled throughout. I wedged the circular carton between my thighs while I drove to thaw it more rapidly around the edges. That way I could wolf it down even faster. I carried a tablespoon in the glove compartment for just such emergencies.

Another pint of ice cream, along with an ample supply of other sugary and salty snack foods, sat in the grocery sacks on the car seat next to me. I had been traumatized at the meeting, I told myself. I needed a little comfort food to help me get over it. It was only a little after noon; I'd just call this my lunch. A person has to eat, you know.

Backhanded inspiration

My social life was nil. What man in his right mind would honestly consider dating a 396-pound woman? And what in heaven's name would I want with a man who *would* consider it? Surely there'd be much more wrong with *him* than with me. The mere logistics of any possible physical or, heaven forbid, *sexual contact*, were beyond my most creative imagination.

In my brain I knew all that, but my heart just couldn't accept I was destined to be irrevocably unlovable.

I constantly fumed, stewed, and sounded off about how

shallow most men were. I ranted and raved how I was the very same person inside whether I was fat on the outside or not. "Where are all the quality men?" I lamented.

I must have sounded pretty pitiful. Downright pathetic. If I had been brutally honest with myself, I would have taken a good long look in the mirror and understood that I wasn't exactly presenting the most salable package. If I had been a guy, I wouldn't have wanted to date me either.

So I turned to the Internet for my "love fix." Every evening I entered chat-rooms under assumed names and personas and got some kind of perverted gratification from being able to dupe the more gullible men purportedly looking for a lasting love via cyberspace.

I described myself as having hair the color of sunlight dancing in the forest, eyes like warm milk chocolate, and a smile that could heat up the coldest winter night. When pressed for a more detailed account, I said I had an hourglass figure with time to spare for the right guy.

It was innocent fun, I told myself—all fantasy—and surely no one really *believes* any of this stuff.

But every once in a while I let one of those presumably gullible men I corresponded with get to know a little bit about the real me.

Ken was one of those men. Ken lived in Ohio. He was geographically safe enough—I'd never have to meet him. He was my age, smart, and he laughed at my jokes. Best of all, Ken was also obese. He understood. At 6'3" and approximately 430 pounds, Ken was well aware of the trials and tribulations of trying to have a "real life" relationship.

The Internet was just the ticket for long-term communication without having to go out into the world as a couple and be laughed at. It was perfect. We shared our lives without leaving our keyboards. No one pointed and stared, and no one monitored how much we shoved into our mouths while corresponding.

In August, after volumes of emails and a plethora of phone calls, Ken suggested coming for a visit. A visit? Are you kidding me? At first I balked, throwing all kinds of obstacles in the way, but he answered all of my objections, until finally I thought, "*Why not?*" We were friends, after all, and I had checked him out well enough so that I harbored not a nanogram of fear for my well-being.

But timing is everything, and his three-day presence in my home brought a lot of tough issues rushing to the surface. For one, Ken had admitted to being "about 430 pounds." But like me, he hadn't found a scale on which to confirm his exact weight in some time.

When I looked at the bulk he asked his 6'3" frame to carry around, I suddenly realized that although I was 8 or 9 inches shorter than him, if he were correct in his weight estimation, I weighed only 35 or 40 pounds less.

The thought was mind-boggling. Up until then, I had no concept of what I looked like to others. When face-to-face with someone approximately my size (*confirmed by trying to stretch a measuring tape around our respective middles*), I found myself struggling against the horribly sick feelings that instantly welled up into my throat.

I gave Ken my extra-large bed to sleep in and I took the guest room because there was no way in hell he could have fit on the regular-sized bed reserved for guests. My waterbed replacement was a California King mattress, six feet wide and seven feet long, so he could comfortably stretch out without having to lie at an angle.

Yet when I crawled into the guest room bed myself, the mattress and metal bed frame bowed severely under my weight. The whole bed sagged and kind of folded in on itself, leaving my rear end just an inch off the floor.

All night I heard the rhythmic hum of Ken's CPAP breathing machine forcing oxygen into his lungs. Ken, like me, suffered from sleep apnea, but I was not yet "bad enough" to seek medical machinery as an aid to sleeping.

Lying in the next room listening to the machine operate, my imagination brought up all kinds of hospital scenes where respirators were required to do the patients' breathing. I fell asleep thinking of my own difficulties breathing at night and worried about how soon I'd have to rely on a machine for Continuous Positive Airway Pressure.

The first full day of Ken's visit, we went sight-seeing, but after a half dozen or so stops, he asked that we not go to places where he'd have to get out of the car again. It was difficult for him to extract himself from the seat at each stop. He had to grasp the doorframe on each side and kind of roll himself through the opening, while the car listed heavily under his effort.

It's a horrible cliché, but our combined food intake during that long weekend could have easily fed a small army. I'd never had a Binge Buddy before who could eat like I did. We ate most meals in local restaurants, and snacked at home or in the car in between. Food was always within easy reach.

At one place we porked out on huge servings of deep fried chicken and jo-jos, with several side orders of onion rings smothered in tartar sauce. We topped it off by driving to another restaurant just two blocks down the street and indulging in enormous slabs of chocolate fudge cake a la mode for dessert. After that, we spent an hour or so sitting in the car on the ocean beach approach watching others walk along the shore, then picked up a jumbo combination pizza to take home and bake for our dinner.

I rationalized I hadn't really started my weight-loss efforts in earnest, and since this could very well be my last big hurrah, I was going to enjoy it.

On Saturday, I skipped the support group meeting. Why should I leave my out-of-town company to attend a meeting I didn't want to go to anyway? That night we ate buckets of heavily buttered popcorn while we watched videos at home. Although we never said it aloud, we both knew neither one of us could fit into a regular movie theater seat.

I hadn't really thought this bingeing bothered me, but once again, I spent the night doing some serious thinking. By the time Ken left to return to Ohio, I was almost willing to believe I would never eat like that again.

A commitmentphobe makes a major commitment

"So how was your second meeting?" asked my counselor even before I'd gotten myself settled on her couch the next week.

"I couldn't make it. I had company from Ohio."

She pointedly stared at me and said nothing. I wondered how much of our time together was spent in such silence. Pretty expensive silence.

"My friend Ken flew out from Cleveland. You didn't expect me to let him sit and twiddle his thumbs for an hour and a half while I went to some stupid old meeting, did you?"

Without a word, the counselor scooted her chair over to her desk, picked up my check for the current appointment, and tore it in half.

"Hey!" I exclaimed. "What are you doing?!"

"I don't want to work with someone who's not serious about getting help."

My mouth gaped open. I'd heard about tough love, but I had never experienced it firsthand. I was not prepared for the horrific slam of tangible panic against my ribcage.

"You can't do that!" I protested. "That's your income you're throwing away!"

"I thought you were willing to go to any lengths to avoid inpatient treatment." She shrugged. "I don't want to work with someone who doesn't value themselves enough to do even the most basic required footwork."

She stood and headed for the door to usher me out.

"But—But—" I stammered and stalled, hoping to buy myself a little time while my mind reeled. "I went the week before. I already told you I don't belong there. Isn't there anything else I can do instead?"

Pausing with her hand on the doorknob, she shook her head. "No. Meeting attendance is a condition of our continued sessions."

I jumped at the thought this might not be the end of our time together after all. "All right! I give up! I'll do whatever you say! Just don't abandon me!"

Her lips curled up, and I instinctively knew the reason behind her practiced pseudo-smile was not something I was going to like, or readily embrace.

She sat back down before speaking in a soft, soothing tone. "For starters, you must commit to a dozen meetings before you decide whether or not you belong there. You didn't get this way overnight, and it's not going to be resolved overnight. A dozen meetings. That's only three months. One meeting a week. Are you willing to do that?"

I chewed on my lower lip while I thought about this. I'd often avoided making long-term commitments, and three months sounded like an eternity. My integrity was being questioned. I certainly didn't like the hemmed-in feeling I got when I promised to do something I might not choose to follow through on, yet if I didn't agree, I'd be out the door and on my way—forever fat and with no one to blame but myself.

"I've already gone to one meeting," I said. "Does that one count?"

She smiled her enigmatic and highly effective smile again while I contemplated the fact there's only a one-letter difference between "shrewd" and "shrew."

"Twelve meetings," she repeated.

I sighed and rolled my eyes. I considered it a total waste of time to spend 11 more Saturday mornings in the company of strangers spilling their guts about all their piddly little problems, but I cheered up considerably when I thought about having 11 more weekends when I could rationalize picking up a few pints of Ben and Jerry's ice cream on the way home as a reward for my forced attendance.

I released a long, slow breath. "Okay," I finally agreed. "I can do that. Twelve meetings."

Meeting #11

Throughout August and September I showed up, more than a little begrudgingly, to the weekly support group meetings while I continued my counseling sessions. There was more to work on than my weight. I wasn't stupid; I knew my weight was merely the manifestation of much deeper issues. After struggling through years of depression, I had some anger and resentment to work on, and a psychiatrist had diagnosed me with borderline OCD (*obsessive/compulsive disorder*) the previous year.

As a result of that diagnosis, I had taken five different anti-depressants over a period of six months. I felt like the doctor was just throwing darts at the dartboard, hoping one of the meds he landed on would help me. I had gotten sicker with each one. I'd felt constant nausea, and each night was still fraught with sleeplessness. My anxiety level, with accompanying paranoia, climbed higher and higher.

When the doctor suggested I was "serotonin sensitive" and my body was reacting negatively to too much of the "feel good" chemical bombarding it all at once, I gave up, completely defeated. Abruptly quitting all medications, I told myself I would rather be chronically depressed than perpetually stoned.

As far as being OCD, I figured a little of that was actually a *good* thing. After all, OCD was what gave me the tenacity to get through college a year ahead of schedule, finish my master's degree in less than two summers, pay off my car in half the time, and work like a dog worrying a bone to reach the high professional goals I set for myself.

So I now applied this questionable attribute to my counseling. I read the books she lent me from cover to cover and played her cassette tapes on addictions, obsessions, and compulsions continuously in the car. I took my daily vitamins and supplements, and cared for my cat.

But I hadn't begun to diet. I told her I was watching what I ate, but mostly I just watched the food disappear.

"I'm on the seafood diet," I joked. "I see food, I eat it."

Two and a half months later, I had somehow managed to lose about 10 pounds. I have no idea how. At the meetings I heard stories from others about working their individual food plans. A food plan, and not a diet. There were no demands here to follow a specific program. Each of them designed their own method—something they could personally live with forever.

It sounded good, but all my life I had been either "on" or "off" a diet. I couldn't imagine how to go about formulating a lifestyle where I wasn't obsessed with the number of calories or fat grams or carbohydrates or protein or whatever I was supposed to be consuming. Or not consuming. I knew I'd never be able to eat three sensible meals and live my life in between, as some of the support members claimed worked for them.

Compulsive eating is a disease. That much I had learned and accepted—a disease that wanted me dead. It was as much a disease as any other disabling addiction. It was cunning, baffling, and powerful, and I had been born in its clutches. I cursed my "bad genes" and sunk ever lower into the bottomless pit of despair.

On the second Friday night in October, with nothing in my life I could honestly say I was looking forward to, I crawled into bed, pulled the covers over my head and cried myself to sleep. I didn't want to go on living the way things were, but didn't know what to do to change it.

The next morning, since I hadn't mercifully died during the night, I got up, got dressed, and headed out to my support group meeting. Meeting number 11. I only had to go to this meeting, and one more, and then I could say I'd tried it, and it didn't work.

The topic for the day was "Hope." As usual, I hardly listened as others told their stories. Listening to them didn't make me feel the least bit hopeful, and only added more fuel to my own depression. Life sucks, and then you die.

The discussion progressed around the room and soon it was my turn to share. I sat there a long time before opening my mouth. "I don't have any hope," I began in a small, but honest voice. "I can't even remember what hope feels like." I paused. I've always been a very emotional person. I don't know why. I even cry during television commercials for Hallmark cards and Folger's coffee.

Now I tried to keep the tears from starting, but I felt like the little Dutch boy with his finger in the dike, afraid to move, afraid to say another word. Yet something—some power greater than myself—gave me the courage to go on. Something told me I had to do this, to get this out, to accept, acknowledge, and really feel the pain. I was finally ready to admit I was powerless over food.

I grabbed the box of tissues offered and hung onto it with both hands while I forced myself to continue. "I have no hope of ever being a normal size again. I have no hope at all. None. I'm sorry to be such a downer, but I haven't had any hope at all for so long..." My voice trailed off. The other women remained silent witnesses while I thought about what more I wanted, or needed, to say.

"Or joy," I added softly. "I can't honestly remember the last time I felt either hope or joy." I started to sob so hard I really couldn't say another word. I motioned for the next person to go ahead and take her turn while I struggled in vain to get myself under control.

The meeting concluded with the words "Keep coming back," but I knew I was never going back. Never. *Never, never, never, never, never!*

Something to hold on to

Commitment or no commitment, 11 meetings were all I could take. Once again, I dodged the hugs and the after-

meeting chit-chat and bolted for my car. The tires spewed gravel behind me as I hastily drove out of the parking lot. I couldn't get away fast enough. I needed to outrun these unsettling and uncomfortable feelings. I needed to hurry as quickly as possible and stuff them down with my Saturday ritual feeding of Ben and Jerry's ice cream.

The tears kept coming as I sped like a maniac towards the store. I probably shouldn't have been driving—I could hardly see through my tears. The pain ripped through me, cutting deeper and deeper until it was almost unbearable. I pounded on the steering wheel with my fists as I drove, sobbing uncontrollably. Aloud, I shouted, *"God, if you're going to help me, now would be a really good time!"*

And then, for some unexplainable reason, I altered my route. It was difficult for me to imagine *anything* getting between me and my food, but instead of making a beeline directly to the grocery store, I decided to make a quick stop at the post office to pick up my mail. I suppose it was so I could go straight home to eat after shopping with no detours, but I'd never done it that way before.

In amongst the usual assortment of bills and mail order catalogs for jumbo-sized clothing was a greeting card from a woman friend I had not seen or talked to in some time. I recognized the return address, and tore into the envelope as soon as I got back into my car.

The front of the card had a watercolor picture on it of a bouquet of wildflowers. Inside, my friend had written: "Here's something for you to hold on to." The card contained a small, folded-over piece of tag board, the approximate size of a silver dollar. The tiny makeshift package was taped shut all around.

I used a fingernail file to cut through the tape and a flat, polished, purple and white marbled rock dropped into my lap. "Swell," I snidely said aloud, "I can tie this rock around my neck when I jump into the river."

I picked up the rock and rubbed my thumb across the smooth finish. *A worry stone?* I wondered. I turned it over. The hair on the back of my neck stood straight up. Engraved in gold on the other side of the rock was one single word: "Hope."

I looked again at what she'd written: "Something to hold onto." She had sent me Hope. A shudder ran through me and I shook my head in disbelief.

The odds against this happening were astronomical. No way could this particular rock, with this particular message, arrive in my particular mailbox on this particular day. Unless, of course, one happens to believe in the intervention of a Higher Power, a Divine Spirit, the One Mind orchestrating the Universe. God, by any other name. God had used my dear friend to send me a most timely message of Hope.

I've never been one to believe in accidents or coincidence. Absolutely everything happens for a purpose. This purpose rang as loud and clear as a million church bells on Christmas morning.

I drove straight home from the post office and placed my precious rock next to the centerpiece on my dining room table where I would surely see it every time I was headed for the kitchen.

I had not stopped at the grocery store for my food fix after the meeting. I felt no compulsion to eat my customary Saturday pint, or two, of ice cream. For some strange reason, I felt no compulsion to eat anything at all.

My New York cheerleader

That Saturday night was undoubtedly the longest night in recorded history. I hadn't had my ice cream to help me numb the feelings that surfaced during the morning's support group meeting, and I hadn't stuffed myself at dinnertime either. By the wee hours of Sunday morning, I was experiencing the pangs of real hunger, but my nagging fear was food would no longer make my discomfort go away—not even temporarily.

My night had been spent in restless pacing. I felt fragile, uncertain, tentative, and terribly vulnerable. I had the feeling I was precariously balanced on a precipice, and I didn't have any idea which way I was about to fall.

Desperate for some type of human connection, I logged onto the Internet to access the chat rooms. I couldn't stand the isolation another minute. If I wasn't going to turn to food, I'd have to turn to something, or someone. Anyone. From anywhere.

"Send me an angel, God," I prayed as I waited for my computer to boot up. *"I need an angel."*

And God sent me David. Just like that, no questions asked, David appeared on my computer screen and began to chat privately with me.

"What's a nice girl like you doing in a place like this?" David typed.

"What do you know about nice girls?" I countered. "You don't know a thing about me. Not a damn thing." And for once in my life, I let down my guard, got rigorously honest, and told the truth about myself and my disease of compulsive overeating.

David, from New York City. David, who stood 5'4," weighed 130 pounds, and who had never had an issue with being overweight in the 47 years of his entire life, did not cut and run. He listened, asked questions, offered suggestions, and hung right in there.

New York David was the perfect answer to my prayer. He was kind, compassionate, and a good communicator. I poured my heart out to him. I told him all about the devastating burden that had always plagued me. I confessed my true weight. I despaired at feeling useless and unworthy and unlovable. David read my words attentively and typed back thoughtful and appropriate replies.

"Life is hell," I wrote him. "I'm too weary to try again. I'm too weak. I'll never make it. I need moral support twenty-four seven. I don't know if I can go on like this much longer."

"Of course you can," he typed back. "Let me help you."

Help me? I read the screen in disbelief. Why would some stranger want to help me? "What's in it for you?" I queried. "Nobody's that altruistic."

"I work in Human Resource Development," David responded. "You are a very valuable resource. The world needs people like you. I want to help."

I only half believed him. I'd never met anyone as selfless and giving and kind, or at least I'd never been consciously able to recognize such unconditional acceptance. I decided to keep an open mind about his offer of help and take it at face value—at least for the time being.

'Have you overeaten today?" he wrote.

"How could I have overeaten today?" I typed back. "I've been attached to my keyboard for hours."

"Then today is day one," he replied.

His energy and enthusiasm inspired me, and in a matter of days he quickly convinced me his commitment to putting me back on the right path was for real.

"Forward is the only viable direction," he wrote. "The

only reason to look over your shoulder is to see how far you've come. Defeat is not an option."

"You are my New York cheerleader," I wrote. "I will never forget you."

"I won't let you ever forget me," he answered. "I will be right here beside you, every step of the way."

Sunday, October 10, 1999. Ten-ten of ninety-nine. My first full day of abstinence from compulsive overeating. My first full day of committing myself to true recovery.

Eskimos

My counselor gave me another cassette tape to listen to that week. On it was the story of a devout man and an atheist conversing in an Alaskan bar. The atheist tells the devout man he gave God a test, that God had failed him, and that's why he doesn't believe.

The devout man asks what kind of a test the atheist had given God to prove Himself.

"I was about 40 miles north of here on a snowmobile," replied the atheist. "A blizzard came up. I couldn't see more than a few feet in front of me. I got lost. I didn't know which way to go to get home and I didn't have enough gas to wander off in the wrong direction. I began to panic. I got off my snowmobile, got down on my knees in the snow, and prayed to your God. I said, 'God, if you're there, you've got to do something quick, cause you know I'm gonna die here if you don't save me'."

"Well then!" exclaimed the devout man, clapping him on the shoulder. "You must believe! "You're here! You're alive! God must have saved you!"

"Oh hell no," said the atheist, disgustedly shaking his

head. "Your God didn't do a damn thing. Not one damn thing. It was just lucky for me an Eskimo happened along about then and pointed out the right way to go to get back to town!"

I didn't need to be hit with a sledgehammer. The woman who sent me the rock with "Hope" written on it was definitely one of my Eskimos. David was another. In a strange way, my Ohio friend Ken also fit into this category. And my counselor, and the Physician's Assistant who had sent me to her, and perhaps, if I gave them a real chance, perhaps even some of the women in the support group would be there for me too.

Soon I had a sneaking suspicion if I kept my eyes open, I would become acutely aware of the multitude of Eskimos God was sending my way. The people who were showing up at exactly the right time and in exactly the right place to do God's work.

The disease of compulsive overeating wanted me dead. God wanted me to live. I made a conscious decision right then and there—while listening to the cassette as I drove to work—to see what would happen if I turned my will and my life over to the care of God—God, as I understood Him.

Now the real work could begin.

A food plan for life

The first thing I felt I had to do was come up with some kind of eating regime I thought I might be able to stick with for the rest of my life, day in, day out, and with no time off for good behavior.

Diets don't work for a compulsive overeater. I had tried dozens of them. If they worked, I would have found a way years ago to binge and purge through the selective use of random hit-and-miss dieting and maintain a normal weight. Restricting one type of food, or indulging in only a select few, always made me arch my back with resistance. My willful inner child absolutely refused to feel deprived.

The mere idea of "going on a diet" implied that someday I would be "going *off* a diet" and could resume eating as I always had. Being on a diet meant that all I ever thought about were the foods I couldn't have, and the constant cravings had always pushed me over the edge and into the bakery in a matter of days.

By definition, a diet is the "food and drink regularly provided or consumed; habitual nourishment." That was a good place for me to start evaluating what I ate.

If the food had no nutritional value, I decided I probably could go without eating or drinking it. Following that suggestion, the first two things on the chopping block were alcohol and all desserts.

I heard myself cry "foul!" and immediately felt like a poor little picked-on kid. However, I quit kicking and screaming and put on my big girl panties (*no pun intended*). I did stop drinking alcohol, and all but eliminated "covert sugar" by limiting my sugar intake to occasional small amounts of dark chocolate only.

I started revamping my thought process to think of my food intake as the nourishment needed to perform daily activities and nothing more. I had to convince myself food was simply the fuel needed to run the machine.

But I *liked* food. I liked the tastes, the textures, the feeling of satiation after consuming an abundant quantity of my favorites. Food had always been much more than mere nutrition. Eating was a social event, a coping skill, a pastime to alleviate the pain of isolation, loneliness, boredom and unworthiness, just to name a few.

There's a very good reason it's called "comfort food," but instead of being comforted, I now felt terribly distressed whenever I used food to numb my feelings. And that meant I was feeling bad about myself on a daily basis.

I earned enough money I could afford to eat well. When I ate at home, I could be sure no one was watching the quantities consumed. When I ate out, I frequently ate dinner at two different restaurants the same evening. After finishing up at one place, I often drove directly to another location and ordered a whole new meal.

I knew I was safe. I knew I wouldn't run into anyone who had seen me dine at the first place, because no one else ate like I ate, or was sick enough to do what I was doing.

Sometimes I ate an early dinner out and then later at home consumed copious amounts of the groceries I'd purchased the same day. One of my usual habits was to devour an entire frozen pizza supreme as though it were an after-dinner mint, often cutting off hunks and shoving it in my mouth before it was fully cooked.

On too many occasions to count, I ate five or six candy bars or a couple bags of chips, or both, as I stood peering through the oven window, willing the pizza to cook faster.

Clearly, I was "self-medicating" with food. I was living to eat instead of eating to live. And ironically, the way I ate could very well kill me.

At this point, I actually envied alcoholics, drug addicts, and smokers. When they quit drinking or drugging or smoking, they got to quit the activity completely. As in *none*. A compulsive overeater can't just stop eating. At least three times a day, we must consume the very thing that is destroying us. I couldn't imagine a drinker or smoker who could be given one drink or one cigarette three times a day and be able to successfully stick it out for a lifetime with those limitations.

So the food plan I developed would have to be a good one. A very good one.

Over the years, I had read plenty of nutrition and diet books, and had even taken a nutrition class at a local hospital. I knew I needed to get all my food groups every day. I knew the vitamins and minerals that were necessary to maintain optimum health. I knew the measured amounts that constituted a serving. I knew the calorie count of practically everything I'd ever eaten.

I just didn't know if I could stop with the recommended portion sizes. I wasn't sure a half-cup of anything would be able to satisfy me, and that was usually the standard considered a normal "serving" for almost everything.

Regarding food preparation, I knew the nutritional difference between frying and broiling fish and chicken. Sauces and dressings are obviously loaded with extra fat and calories. Intellectually, I knew exactly what to do. Exactly. But it had to be something I could, at least hypothetically, live with forever.

So I examined my lifestyle. I loved eating out; I didn't love cooking. Cooking a gourmet dinner, in my opinion, shouldn't take much more time in the kitchen than pulling back the corner of the plastic wrap to vent the food on the tray before popping it into the microwave. I was a certified "M & M girl"—Microwaves and Menus.

Therefore, I knew I had to design a food plan that incorporated the essence of who I am without having to make what I considered extreme and drastic changes in every other part of life. My plan had to be simple and easy to implement on a day-to-day basis. My battle cry became "K.I.S.S." —Keep It Simple, Stupid. It had to be so easy that following the plan might someday become effortless, and if not effortless, at the very least it had to be a plan that would not involve too much nit-picky, time-consuming, resentment-building effort.

I figured my original weight goal to be somewhere between 158 and 168 pounds. I had pictures of me in that range, and I had been perfectly happy with myself and how I looked. Never mind what those nasty insurance charts said. "Big bones" notwithstanding, some people were just born to be a little curvier. Voluptuous. Softer in spots.

In my dieting experience, I had learned quite a few math formulas. I had learned it takes about 10 calories per pound of weight to maintain the weight of a person who is not very active. In other words, to maintain my 396 pounds, I must have been consuming approximately 3,960 calories per day. Maybe even a few less, since I was extremely sedentary.

It takes a lot of food to add up to 3,960 calories, but I knew I often crammed in another 2,000 or more just before bedtime, on top of everything I'd already eaten that day.

To lose one single pound, a person has to cut 3,500 calories from their maintenance number. That means to lose a pound per week, a person has to cut out 500 calories per day. For two pounds a week, they cut 1,000 per day, and for three pounds a week, 1,500 fewer calories must be eliminated from each day's usual intake.

Theoretically, consuming 2,400 calories a day should initially give me a 3-pound weekly weight loss. But I knew I'd never be able to lose much weight at 2,400 calories a day. After all, 2,400 calories, using the same formula as before, would support a 240-pound person, and that wasn't an ideal weight either.

The old "diabetic's diet" recommended 1200 calories a

day. There are "new" diet groups out there today that are based roughly on that same 1200 limit, along with elimination of covert sugars, most carbohydrates, and the majority of wheat products. Twelve hundred calories would have equaled starvation for a woman my size.

About then, the numbers began baffling me, so I decided to tackle the problem from another angle.

Instead of focusing on the number of calories I had to cut from my life in order to lose pounds, I calculated how many calories I would be eating once I arrived at my targeted goal weight.

I decided to "feed" the 150-pound woman living within me. (*I chose 150 because it was a nice round number to work with.*) To feed this woman, if she didn't exercise at all, would mean eating approximately 1500 calories a day. If I continued to feed a 150-pound woman, I rationalized, sooner or later I would *be* a 150 pound woman. Or darn close to it.

The idea had immediate appeal, and a sing-song chant began running around inside my head. Over and over I repeated my new mantra: *Feed the woman you want to see. Feed the woman you want to be.*

But 1500 calories didn't sound like much more than 1200, and it sure didn't seem like enough to eat. It might be just a tad too strict, too rigid, and with no built-in margin of error. Was I setting myself up for failure yet again?

I talked it over with New York David. "So how about cutting yourself just a tiny bit slack?" he asked me. "How about setting a *range* of calories you can commit to live with, day in and day out?"

A range sounded like a great idea! I took his advice and set a daily target of 1500 to 2000 calories. The parameters were a little loose, but I felt comfortable with that latitude. I thought there was now enough flexibility within my food plan to allow me some wiggle room to maneuver without guilt or shame—no "all or nothing" caveat.

But I still didn't want to be "dieting." I still wanted to eat whatever types of food I wanted to eat each day. I decided to limit quantity, and nothing more.

It was all about making good choices. Therefore, if I *chose* to eat four maple bars, then I would have to *choose* to call them dinner. Not a sound decision, but I didn't want to have to say a flat "No" to any specific food. I knew I probably *wouldn't* trade maple bars for dinner, but I wanted to know that if I really, really wanted to, I could, and that I wouldn't be throwing out my entire program if I slipped up and did just that.

Next I made a list of my favorite restaurants and the things I most enjoyed ordering. Broccoli Chicken and a little steamed rice at the Chinese place. Fish, baked potato and salad bar, if one was available, were staples of several places on my list. And I'd been eating quite a variety of Subway sandwiches (*sans cheese and mayo*) long before I ever heard of Jared Fogle.

I counted the calories in each of my coveted restaurant offerings. Knowing how much I craved a substantial meal in the evening, I carefully rationed my calories at breakfast and lunch so I could have a larger, more fulfilling, dinner.

Breakfast became a cup of light yogurt (*100 calories*) and often a piece of fruit (*80-100 calories*). Mid-morning I had a V-8 juice (*70*). At lunch, because I craved the crunching, I usually grabbed a full bag of low-fat microwave popcorn (*225 for a whole bag!*). Occasionally, lunch consisted of a canned "liquid meal" (*200*) or a lean microwave entree (*270-330*).

By the end of most workdays I had eaten between 400

and 650 calories. That left me a full 1000, give or take, for dinner. I recorded my food groups each day and made sure I was eating a reasonably-balanced diet.

I became "The Queen of Rounding Off." For a cup of vegetables I wrote down 50 calories. A whole raw fruit or two cups of any peeled and cubed fruit was now a flat 100. Bread, whatever kind, 100 per slice. Rice, a whopping 200 a cup. A plain, average-sized baked potato put another 120 down in my food diary. Meats usually ranged between 50 and 60 an ounce, and four ounces of meat, about the size of a deck of cards, wasn't going to satisfy me even if it *was* the recommended portion size, so I always allotted myself six to eight ounces of protein at dinnertime.

I packed my freezer from top to bottom with low-fat, low-calorie, pre-made meals. There were so many to choose from! Lean Cuisine, Healthy Choice, Smart Ones, Budget Gourmet, Weight Watchers and many more. Although I admit that most nights I ate more than one such meal, and sometimes three or four, I knew I wasn't doing myself any harm as long as I stuck to the basics of my nutritionally sound food plan.

For good measure, I took vitamin supplements. Vitamins A, C, E and selenium came together as an "antioxidant" and I took extra calcium as well. I was sure my inner 150-pound woman, soon to be approaching menopause, would appreciate the extra calcium.

With my food plan firmly in place by the end of the second week, all I had to do now was stick to it. And for that, as much as I hated to admit it, I could use some outside assistance.

Garnering more support

I called and/or emailed my New York Cheerleader on a daily basis, clinging to the belief that by some long-distance sleight-of-hand magic miracle, he could keep me from falling back into the pattern of compulsive overeating. And perhaps he did.

Each day David asked about my food intake, listened to my crisis du jour, and figuratively patted me on the back while using his other hand to hold tight to one of mine.

"The man must be a saint!" I thought time and again. How he managed to be so upbeat, positive and supporting through those first few weeks is beyond me. I began to refer to him not only as my "Eskimo" and "Cheerleader," but also as my "New York Angel."

As much as I didn't want to, I kept attending the support group. During the introduction to each meeting, a brief preamble ends with the words "You are not alone." Well, it sure *felt* like I was alone at three in the morning when I awoke with my empty stomach trying to gnaw its way through my backbone.

At 3 a.m. west coast time, it's still only 6 a.m. in New York, and I was at least a little sensitive about David's sleep schedule. So I went back online and looked for chat rooms where I could find sympathetic friends who knew what I was going through. I was never disappointed. At any time of day or night I was able to touch base with other obsessive/compulsive people all around the world.

It didn't matter what their specific addictions were, when you're working toward recovery, it's any port in a storm. The lifelines they threw my direction got me past many potential relapses. And these people, nameless and faceless though they be, cared enough to encourage me to keep attending the local support group and look for someone there who could be my special link, up close and personal, to stick with the program.

The following Saturday, I took another good look at the women seated around the room. I knew by now that no two people had the same food plan. We represented all shapes and sizes and levels of commitment. A few of the women were at goal and successfully maintaining their weight. *That's where I want to be*, I thought.

That thought stuck with me throughout the following week. I began considering one woman in particular to be my special weight-loss confidant—the woman who had greeted me at the door at my first meeting. How did she get to her goal, and how had she learned how to *stay* at goal?

The nagging idea that I wanted what she had finally prompted me to call her between meetings. "You have a clavicle," I said. "I *think* I have one too, but it's been so long since I've seen it… Can you, will you, help me?"

The one woman I chose to bare my soul to, the one woman I risked showing my vulnerability to, the one woman I most admired in the group—turned me down flat.

She had too much on her plate, she said—she was spread too thin (*no puns intended*). She was involved in a lot of activities other than this group and she didn't feel she would be able to give me the kind of quality time she thought I'd need.

I thanked her for her honesty, hung up, and went straight to the kitchen. I stood in front of the open fridge and cried. I'd been rejected. I felt unworthy and unlovable. I wanted something to help me numb these troubling feelings. *I wanted food.*

But I didn't eat. I still don't know why, but I didn't. I got out a diet soda instead. I opened one of the books I'd gotten at the support meeting and began to read.

At that moment, I knew God was watching over me. *Everything will be fine*, He now seemed to tell me. I have my counselor, I have NY David, I'm attending meetings, I can surely do this without having one more person to lean on.

It never occurred to me to call another woman in the group. I had done a lot of soul searching before calling this first one, and I knew she was the "kick butt" sort of woman who would take no prisoners and not cut me, or my self-created food plan, any undermining slack. She was exactly the type of woman I sought—one who could support me without being too soft. I knew what I needed, and I didn't need any mollycoddling.

I wasn't about to stick my neck out like that again. Her answer had been "No." I would accept that and go on working my program by myself. I could do it, I *had been* doing it, and I certainly didn't need to eat to cope with this little disappointment.

The surprising thing was, I *didn't* eat over it. Not that day, and not the next. When I'd randomly opened the used book to put some space between my food thoughts and actions, it had opened to the section on "acceptance." Perhaps the previous owner had creased the page with numerous readings, or perhaps it was my Higher Power guiding me to just the thing I needed at that moment.

As I began to read, I remembered another friend telling me to "Celebrate the 'No's," and rest assured God had greater plans for me, if I would just surrendered my will and my life and put my trust in Him.

So I prayed for acceptance. But I still didn't find the reserves inside me to call anyone else to be my support buddy. And just a little over a week later, the woman I had first phoned called me back and asked if I still wanted her to work with me.

I went to bed that night with one prevalent thought echoing inside me: God is good.

Dream it; believe it

"What do you really want?" asked David during one of my more panicky phone calls. "Do you really want to eat everything you can get your hands on, or do you have some long-term goals that overeating right this very minute will not help you attain?"

His question stopped me in my tracks. It didn't take me a full heartbeat to start listing the things I dreamed about having in my life.

"I want to be HWP," I told him. "In the personal ads that stands for height/weight proportionate. I figure for me that's somewhere between 158 and 168. I won't be a skinny-minnie, but at that weight I'll be able to hold my own with a woman of any size."

"And this is important to you?" he asked.

"Yes!" I replied. "There's an awful lot of competition out there—for jobs, for men, for respect in general. I'm tired of coming in last because of my size. I don't want to be stared at, or laughed at, or pitied. I want to be judged solely on the quality of my character and not the size of my clothing—"

"You have a dream…" David interjected, in what I misconstrued as a decidedly condescending tone.

"Don't you dare laugh at me!" I heard my voice go up at least one full octave. "Don't you, of all people, laugh at me! You're my rock, David, not the guy who's going to throw them at me!"

"I wasn't laughing honey," he said. "I just wanted to get you down from that soapbox before you got a nosebleed."

I readily admitted I had been off and running on a bit of a diatribe. I took a deep breath and reconsidered his question. So what *did* I really want?

To be HWP, yes, that was definitely high on the list. And to have the professional respect I knew I deserved. I wasn't able to separate those two thoughts, so for the time being, I let them sit right there together.

In the back of my closet hung a bright blue blouse—electric blue—and I wanted to wear that blouse again someday. But there again, I was basing my ultimate happiness solely on a specific size of clothing.

As I had told my support group friend, I wanted to see my clavicle. I wanted my health and fitness back. I wanted to be able to walk a couple miles on the beach without stopping to gasp for air. I even dreamed of participating in "The Great Columbia River Crossing," an annual 10K walk across the imposing Megler-Astoria Bridge.

I wanted to fit comfortably into any movie theater seat.

I didn't want to worry about having to ask for a seatbelt extender in an airplane, and I wanted the lap tray to be able to come all the way down to a flat position without hanging up on my belly. I wanted the people assigned to the seats beside me not to react with horror when they saw whom they'd be sitting next to for the duration of the flight.

I wanted to be able to go out for a cup of coffee and not have to check first to see if the table and bench were bolted to the wall or floor. I had suffered the embarrassment of not fitting into the booths at more than one local restaurant and I never wanted to face that humiliation again.

These things I shared with David. Tangible things. The physical manifestations of losing a great deal of weight.

Yet there were plenty of other things I wanted. Some things were hard to put words to, and some things weren't very pretty.

I wanted revenge. I wanted to "get even" with all the people who had ever discounted me because of my size. Men, mostly. I wanted to become instantly gorgeous, then flaunt my beauty in front of them and make them eat their hearts out for having once rejected me.

"When you've truly recovered," said my support group buddy, "you won't feel the need to do those things."

Maybe not, I grudgingly agreed. But for the time being, those were the kinds of thoughts that helped keep me motivated.

And although it might sound silliest of all coming from a woman who weighed nearly 400 pounds, what I wanted most was to wear a sparkling long red dress and swing dance with David in a New York nightclub.

"We can do that honey," said David without the slightest hesitation when I shared this dream with him. "Buy the dress; we'll go dancing whenever you're ready."

CHAPTER III:
FIFTY POUNDS DOWN

Willpower vs. won't power

I wonder if hereditary or environmental factors are more to blame for an Obsessive/Compulsive Disorder. Is it in the genes or is it learned behavior? Is it something that lives deep within my DNA, or did I pick it up by watching my mother fanatically try to keep an immaculate house with four small children underfoot? No matter. The point is I'm quite certain I could be at least a runner-up as the poster child for OCD.

Although I never succumbed to excessive hand-washing, or refused to step on any sidewalk cracks (*both exhibited by Jack Nicholson in the movie "As Good As It Gets"*), there is no doubt I suffer to some degree from uncontrollable obsessive thoughts and actions.

Perhaps it's the result of being slightly superstitious as a kid. Don't walk under ladders. Watch out for black cats crossing your path. Lift your feet when the car goes over the railroad tracks. If a bird flies in the window, someone's going to die. If you set your shoes on the table, someone's going to die. If you don't hold your breath and walk fast enough to get to the next corner before the car coming up behind you does, someone's going to die.

Fixations on thoughts like these are childhood fodder

for the adult OCD victim. It's an all or nothing mentality. Black or white. Yes or no. On or off. There's no middle ground whatsoever. He loves me; he loves me not.

For years I replayed each entire day while I laid awake in the middle of the night. I planned my next encounter with certain people I felt had wronged me, or with those whom I wanted to keep from wronging me. I wrote voluminous letters in my mind, championing my newest crusade, or defending some alleged sleight.

I lost so much sleep dwelling on things I had no control over I joked about my epitaph reading: "The wheel's still turning, but the hamster's dead."

A few years prior to beginning my weight-loss journey, I'd sought medical help for my disturbing and relentless thought patterns. The doctor confirmed what I had known all along: Serious clinical depression, and borderline OCD. He prescribed several medications to help short-circuit and re-program my brain waves.

But some of us aren't destined to get relief from chemical remedies. The pills made me sicker than I had been without them. The doctor switched medications. I got sicker. He gave me another and another and yet another prescription.

I began to suspect he was choosing my meds by throwing darts at a dartboard. I had pills lined up across the bathroom counter with post-it notes telling me what time to take each one. The top of my dresser resembled a pharmaceutical display. I took pills for depression, pills for OCD, and pills to combat the inability to keep the first pills down. I was so ill by now nausea was my constant companion. I carried an assortment of salty crackers with me like a pregnant woman during her first trimester.

I could barely go to work each day, yet work was the

only place I felt safe. I was needed at work, and I knew I was still doing a reasonably good job doing what I was trained to do.

I also knew that away from work I was just going through the motions of living. I came home each day and collapsed on the couch. Telling myself I was eating to keep the nausea under control had resulted in my rapidly gaining more weight. It got so bad that I seriously considered suicide. I doubted I would ever get better, and I didn't think I could go on living from pill-to-pill like this much longer.

As a last-ditch effort at understanding what was happening to me, I went back to my Physician's Assistant. She suggested that perhaps I had a "serotonin sensitivity" and that too much of the "feel good chemical" dumped into my system all at once was more than my body could handle. She'd suggested weaning me onto the medications more slowly.

Instead, I metaphorically stomped my foot and arched my back. And then I abruptly stopped taking any meds at all. I simply flushed them down the toilet that very day. I decided then and there that I would rather be depressed and dealing with OCD than be stoned all the time, sick to my stomach, and wandering around in a semi-self-destructive haze. It was an irresponsible and drastic action. It could easily have killed me. I am grateful it did not.

So now, a few years after my sojourn into anti-depressants, as I began the oh-so-slow journey back from morbid obesity, I understood why my squirrel-cage thoughts revolved constantly around food. How much had I already eaten today? What more could I eat and still stay on my plan? How many calories did I have left and still available to consume? How could I eat enough at dinner to feel satisfied and yet stick with the program? Would I be able to abstain from compulsive eating until I could find sanctuary in my bed for the night?

I kept a running calorie tabulation in my day planner. I wondered time and again what "normal" people thought about all day if they weren't obsessing about food. Did they actually not worry about what they were going to eat at their next meal? Did they really "forget to eat" when they were caught up in other activities? What might it feel like to "let go" of the control I attempted to grasp so tightly?

I recited the Serenity Prayer 30 or 40 times a night: "God, grant me the serenity to accept the things I cannot change, the courage to change the things I can, and the wisdom to know the difference."

Only the thing was, I honestly didn't know if I *could* change this behavior. I didn't know if I *could* keep from overeating. I didn't know if I *could* stop the runaway train of thoughts from derailing my whole program. Was I doomed to being obese the rest of my life? Should I "accept" that idea with serenity? Where was I supposed to get this elusive "*Wisdom* to know the difference"? And the scariest of all: Did I *really* want my life to be "different?"

I kept going to the support group meetings. I read the literature. I called my support group buddy every day, and I made phone calls to others who, like me, were valiantly striving to walk the walk. I wrote in my journal. I reached out through email. And I tenaciously stuck to my food plan.

It was one meal, one moment, one mouthful, one MORSEL at a time. I lived in constant fear I would be too mentally weak to stick to my food plan, no matter how generous the latitude I'd given myself when I developed it.

By the barest of threads, by sheer will power—or maybe that's "won't" power—and with determination and guts and lots and lots of outside support along with my tears, the days in the success column slowly added up.

Broasted chicken and the banishing bra

But sometimes even "won't power" just doesn't stand a chance. Sometimes even the firmest of vows needs a very timely booster shot. And sometimes, all that stands between you and one hell of a deep-fried binge is a little Yankee ingenuity.

On a sunny Saturday afternoon, within an hour after attending my weekly support group meeting, I stood before the open refrigerator, pondering my food choices for the day. I'd already had my usual yogurt breakfast, my mid-morning V-8 juice break, and now it was time for a healthy low-calorie lunch.

But today there was nothing in the fridge that appealed to me. I closed the door and peered into the cupboard. Nothing too exciting there, either. What I *really* wanted, I realized, was broasted chicken from the local bar. Nowhere on earth could you find broasted chicken that tasted any better, and the more I thought about it, the more my salivary glands kicked into high gear. Before long, I realized I *had* to have that chicken.

I added up my calories for the day: I was perched and primed at only 170 measly energy units. That gave me a whopping 1330 to mess with, but it had to include lunch *and* dinner. Never mind that I'd be through eating for the day by 2 p.m. and that I'd most likely be ravenous again by 6 or 7 o'clock, I knew what I wanted, and I wanted it *NOW*.

An order of half a broasted chicken was one humongous breast, thigh, wing and drumstick. And of course, there were jo-jos that came with it. Jo-jos and ranch dressing. By carefully manipulating the numbers, I could estimate, with a straight face, the calorie count of that meal coming in at right around 1800 calories.

Eighteen hundred and 170 was 1970. Well, gee! Nineteen-seventy was still within my food plan's upper "limit" of 2000 per day! My target goal was 1500, but I had made a promise that I would not beat myself up if I stayed below 2000 calories in any one day. I could taste the first bite of that scrumptious chicken already.

And then a funny thing happened. Not funny as in "ha-ha," but funny as in very, *very* peculiar. To this day I can only attribute what happened to a power greater than myself, and with a much more stubborn backbone.

As I rushed to pull on my tennis shoes, I debated whether or not to call ahead so they could have my coveted food, which I knew took 20 minutes to prepare even if there weren't any orders ahead of me, ready to pick up and take out the moment I arrived. No way was I going to eat it *there*, where others could watch me wolf it down. I planned on going to the beach approach to eat in peaceful solitude— also known as "eating in secret."

"Solitude?" "Secret?" I heard a little voice ask. "Just what kind of a sane food plan justifies sneak eating?"

That little voice, my fledgling food conscience, was becoming a tad bit annoying. More often than not, that little voice was messing up some previously very enjoyable eating experiences.

It's not sneak eating, I thought to myself. *It's legal food on my legal food plan.*

"Yeah, right," said the little voice in a tone I previously thought was reserved solely for snotty seventh graders.

I stopped grappling with my shoelaces, and sat totally

still for a moment on the living room steps. *What are you really up to?* I asked myself.

"You're not going to like the answer," said my little voice.

So what shall I do about it?

"Put all your bras into the washing machine."

I beg your pardon?

"You know you won't leave the house without a bra on," said my little voice. "Do what you need to do to keep from going out and beginning what could turn out to be the ominous start of a multi-day binge. You have no idea where this one indulgent meal could lead you. Do the right thing here, girlfriend."

I cringed. *No! I want my broasted chicken! I'll only eat the chicken! I'll skip the jo-jos and the ranch dressing! Please!*

The little voice was silent.

It's difficult to argue with silence.

Still sitting on the carpeted steps, I sighed in defeat. I kicked off my shoes. I stood up and pulled my shirt over my head. I unhooked my 52 double F bra and took it off right where I was standing. I walked into the utility room. "This is crazy," I said aloud.

But crazy or not, when I threw my bra into the washer, turned the water on and went into the bedroom to retrieve my other two trusty undergarments, I knew in my heart it was the right thing to do. Throwing my bras into the washer banished any thought of leaving the house, just as my little voice said it would.

And when you stop long enough to listen to your little voices, you become more willing to go to any lengths to stick with your food plan. You're halfway home. So I dropped the rest of my laundry in with my bras, added detergent, and picked up the phone to call New York

David.

I knew David would get a kick out of this story, and I loved to hear him laugh.

Maggie and Miki and Me

"Relatives you're born with, friends you get to choose." So states a wise old Russian proverb.

I met Maggie in 1974, during my last year of college. Monday through Friday for the duration of fall term, we commuted 35 miles each way to our practice teaching classes. Somewhere along the road we became lifelong friends.

I met Miki a little over a dozen years later when she first came to teach in our school district. Although we worked in different buildings, we took some of the same inservice classes and we were very much alike.

Besides teaching, Maggie and Miki and I shared another commonality. We had all had a lifelong struggle with food. When I'd last seen Maggie, she was a little over 300 pounds. Miki had been hovering somewhere close to 250.

In early November, about a month into my commitment to my food plan, I began to reach out to friends like these from whom I had inadvertently pulled away as my weight skyrocketed up near 400 pounds. Now I was ready for their support. They "knew me when." Swallowing my pride, I made contact.

I wrote Maggie a long email and told her exactly what I was doing. She wrote back that she had begun attending Weight Watchers the previous March. "It's all new," she replied. "It's not like when we were in college. It's a points system now. Every food has a point value. You eat until you've used up your allotted points for the day."

"Isn't that just like counting calories and/or balancing food groups?" I asked her.

"Oh, I could *never* count calories," she replied.

When I called Miki, I discovered she, too, had begun a weight loss program. She had been following the Prism program since June. "It's based on roughly 1200 calories a day," she explained, "and I'm not eating sugar at all."

"Twelve hundred calories a day and no sugar sounds like the old diabetic diet."

"I suppose it's similar," Miki agreed. "Everything old is new again."

I wondered if there was something in the air, or in the water, or maybe in the alignment of the planets, that the three of us would all begin taking better care of our bodies within just a few months of each other. Maybe it was the onset of middle age. Or maybe it was just because it was now *time* to make a change.

I shared Miki's success with Maggie and vice versa. "We're going to make it," I wrote. "All three of us. I can feel it in my bones. It doesn't matter what plan or program we follow, it only matters that we are 100% committed to sticking with it."

The others concurred.

My support structure had now increased by two. Two strong, intelligent, fun-loving, capable, competent and dedicated women.

Giving thanks for broccoli and other green things

Six weeks into my commitment I butted up against the holiday specifically dedicated to stuffing oneself with stuffing. Not even in my wildest imagination could I fathom living through the fourth Thursday in November without eating to excess.

Understandably terrified, I knew I couldn't trust myself to go anywhere *near* my family of origin; there were way too many land mines to navigate. Dealing with life-long familial issues while precariously clinging to my fledgling food plan was too much to ask. I didn't have enough time invested in this new lifestyle to feel comfortable not using food to medicate around my relatives.

It may sound simplistic, but all my life I had "coped" with the family drama by overeating. Not wanting to get sucked back into my old, ineffective coping skills when I was just getting my life back on track, I talked it over with friends in my support group. Putting me first, and practicing good self-care, I politely declined the invitations to "go north" for the holidays.

I considered going out to a local restaurant, one where there *wasn't* going to be an all-you-can-eat buffet, and ordering a simple turkey dinner. My mouth watered profusely as I scanned the newspaper. Each restaurant advertised their take on the traditional national food fest. I shook my head to clear my thinking. No, restaurant dining wasn't the answer either.

Well, I could always stay home and eat the infamous Hungry Man's Turkey TV Dinner. Or maybe two or three of them. Or maybe I could forgo the actual dinner and head right for dessert. I could get a deep-dish pumpkin pie and eat the whole darn thing and probably be none the worse for wear—as long as I promised myself that would be *all* I'd eat that day.

Of course Miki sympathized. She was the designated cook for her family, yet she was determined to stick with her Prism food plan. She suggested I have dinner at her house so we could encourage each other. I declined, saying it was a "family time," she would be surrounded by her own relatives, her house was rather small, I wouldn't feel comfortable crashing in, and besides, I didn't want her thinking I was there to be her food monitor.

She took my words at face value and told me the invitation would remain open even if I woke up on Thursday and had suddenly changed my mind.

On top of everything else, my car wasn't working properly and I was afraid to stray too far from home. Thoughts about heading down the Oregon coast for a couple days were dismissed as that geographical escape plan was no longer an option.

I lapsed into a bad case of self-pity. Poor, poor me. Poor, poor me can't eat like a normal person and therefore poor, poor me can't enjoy Thanksgiving. Poor, poor me.

Thanksgiving eve my old friend Pat from Port Angeles called and told me he was on his way "to the ocean." He said to expect him the next day around noon. I told him not to come, there was no food in the house, and I was going to treat it as just an ordinary day around here. He said not to worry about fixing anything, we'd wing it when he arrived.

So the next morning I got showered and dressed after all. My back-up plan had been to stay in bed all day and intermittently read and watch football. I hadn't quite figured out the food aspect yet. My friend Pat forced me to shake off some of my despairing thoughts. I found myself actually looking forward to his visit.

Pat arrived bearing food: Two turkey and cranberry sauce sandwiches from the local bakery. "It's against the law not to eat turkey on Thanksgiving," he explained. "There's no mayonnaise on yours."

I looked at my friend a long time before I said a single word. I could have laughed, I could have cried, I could have slathered my own light mayonnaise all over my sandwich and devoured it in three bites.

But I didn't. I didn't need to. God had sent His emissary to help me stick with my food plan. Another Eskimo.

And I suddenly knew I could enjoy a traditional Thanksgiving without overeating. The day didn't have to be about food. It didn't have to be about massive gluttony. It didn't have to be about stuffing myself until I lapsed into a sick food coma. I suddenly knew, really *knew*, deep down in my toes, I didn't have to eat like that ever again. A power greater than myself had miraculously taken charge.

Pat understood. He'd made an over four hour drive on my behalf simply because he understood. I felt an overwhelming sense of serenity and gratitude.

I took both sandwiches from him, put them into the refrigerator, and allowed myself the first genuine smile of the day as I picked up the phone.

"Miki?" I asked, when my calorie-counting compadre answered my call, "Exactly what time is dinner, would you like me to bring a cheeseless broccoli casserole, and is there room for one more guest besides me at the table?"

Promptly at 2 p.m., we all bowed our heads and gave gratitude for loving, understanding, compassionate friends.

And not one of us overate.

Singing the car buying blues

My car was nine years old and had over 130,000 hard-earned miles on it. The trips to the repair shop had become alarmingly frequent. On Thanksgiving eve my vehicle had refused to restart after I shut it off at the gas station.

It was time to buy something new, but I was dragging my feet. I had purchased my Honda Accord in 1991 simply because it was the only car I could find at the time I could fit into. Now I was 30 or 40 pounds heavier. I was terrified I wouldn't be able to find anything I could safely drive and stay within my budget.

"Get a Toyota," said my friend Pat. "You'll fit in a Camry, I'd bet on it."

I didn't want a Toyota. I didn't want to have to buy any car at all. I didn't want to go through the humiliation of pulling onto a new car lot and having all the lean and hungry salesmen look me over and run the other way, sure I was there just to waste their opportunity to make a sale with a more...uh..."viable" customer.

But I also didn't want to put any more money into the car I had. It was time. And when it's time, if we pay the least bit of attention, an opportunity always presents itself.

My "opportunity" arrived in the form of a flyer enclosed in the newspaper I'd purchased to check out the day after Thanksgiving "Black Friday" sales. Naturally, because there is only one Divine Mind at work in the entire Universe, the flyer advertised a Toyota sale in Longview— a "neighboring community" 75 miles up the Columbia River.

I took a deep breath, then located the title to my car, emptied the trunk and glove box, wiped off the dashboard and vacuumed under the seats. When I arrived in Longview I ran it through a car wash.

Pangs of separation anxiety began to take hold as I neared the car lot. My hot little metallic cranberry red Honda had served me well for nine years. I loved this car! The tales it could tell! And yet, I knew there was very little "get up and go" left in it. Still, I balked at the thought of giving up that part of my "youth."

Once at the Toyota dealership, it went pretty much as I'd envisioned. As I got out of my car, a dozen circling sharks huddled and conferred and shoved from among them a very young and obviously inexperienced salesman. He cautiously approached me, wiping his clammy hand on his slacks before extending it. He asked what kind of car I was looking for.

"Did you lose the coin toss?" I couldn't help asking.

He looked bewildered.

"The joke's on them," I said, motioning to the group of salesmen next to the office. "I am here to buy a car today. Do you want to sell me a car?"

He laughed nervously. "I haven't sold a car all month," he confessed.

It was November 28.

"Then today's your lucky day," I said. "Show me a car I can fit into without having to wedge my stomach against the steering wheel and I'll buy it."

He thought I was kidding. I wasn't.

I figured I'd need to get a 2-door because I thought the wider door would give me easier access to the driver's seat. I also wanted a 2-door because a 4-door was indicative (*at least in my mind*) of middle-aged people with families, who naturally *needed* a 4-door car.

But for some unknown reason, taking away two doors adds a great deal more to the selling price of a vehicle. And the first few cars the salesman showed me were much more money than I could comfortably afford. In other words, all the 2-door Toyotas were way beyond my budget. Reluctantly, I asked him to show me a 4-door model.

The first 4-door car he showed me was not any color I ever would have chosen. Not in this lifetime. It was gray.

Secret Service gray. A plain, nondescript, milquetoast, conservative 4-door Camry, and certainly not representative of the woman inside me who was screaming her head off for a fire-engine-red corvette convertible or some equally bright color of a hot Mustang GT.

But this was the car listed in the newspaper sale flyer. He called it "the ad car." I called it "the bait to get me here car," since there were no other cars of this make and model and price available. So gray it was. Take it or leave it. It fit my budget, and with any luck, I would be able to fit inside and still manipulate the steering wheel.

The kid, despite his lack of years, was no dummy. He reached inside and adjusted the steering wheel as high as it would go and then moved the driver's seat all the way back before he held the door open for me.

I got in. So far, so good, but I couldn't quite reach the pedals. I tentatively moved the electric seat forward until I could just touch the accelerator with ball of my right foot.

I laid my hand flat on my stomach and rubbed it up and down. The back of my hand rubbed against the edge of the steering wheel. I tried to move the seat back just a little, but found even the slightest adjustment left me pressing the gas and brake pedals with only the very tips of my toes.

I moved the seat forward again until there was less than a half-inch of space between my stomach and the steering wheel; I could barely breathe without bumping against it. The young salesman gently closed my door and got in on the passenger side. He began pointing out the various dials and functions on the dashboard.

The trunk latch and gas cap release levers were on the floor next to the driver's seat. I couldn't begin to reach either of them without opening the door and leaning more than half way out of the vehicle.

"Before you go any further," I said, "I better see if I can actually drive this thing." I started the car and drove it carefully off the lot and onto the road. I had lived in Longview years before, so I didn't need him to tell me where to turn to get to the freeway. The car handled fine, and I returned to the sales lot without incident.

Then, and only then, did I reach around me for the seatbelt. I pulled the strap out as far as my arm extended and attempted to wrap it around me.

"Do you want a little help with that?" asked the salesman.

"Do you come with the car to help me fasten the seatbelt every time I drive it?" I replied.

He blushed and sat still while I blindly wrestled with the buckle. When it finally snapped into place, I heaved a great sigh of relief.

"Now let's see if I can get out of here," I said, fumbling for the release button. "And we can go sharpen up that pencil of yours."

He grinned, and I grinned back.

I drove almost halfway home in my plain, nondescript, 4-door conservative gray Camry before I took a good look in the rearview mirror. The woman who looked back was a middle-aged, morbidly obese, milquetoast middle-school teacher. I pulled the car to the side of the road and sobbed.

I allowed myself to sit in my grief and fully experience it. Then I got out my pen and added a hot, racy new sports car on my list of ultimate weight-loss rewards. I'd forgo the idea of a red Corvette for another Mustang. I'd had three Mustangs in the past, and I fervently hoped there was still at least one more waiting in my future.

Finding the willingness to be me

Between Thanksgiving and Christmas I decided to take my first turn at chairing a support group meeting. The leadership rotated on a volunteer basis, and after attending without fail for four and a half months, I finally "womaned-up" and took the hot seat.

As I read the preamble to the meeting aloud, I was suddenly struck by one of those metaphorical thunderbolts. What flashed before my eyes was the word "honest."

I realized I hadn't been the least bit honest at any of these meetings. Not one. I hadn't gotten down and dirty. I wasn't willing to bare the part of me that needed the most repair. I was a fake and a fraud.

There were women attending this meeting who knew that. Some of them had known from the very beginning, but respecting my decision, had not blown my cover. I was grateful for that, but now it also added to my sense of sudden deep remorse and painful guilt.

Living in a small town, teaching in a small school, writing for a small town newspaper, I hadn't wanted to tarnish my self-presumed "reputation" by being honest about my identity at these meetings. So at the very first meeting I'd attended, I had made up a name to use.

After all, I rationalized, what possible difference could it make? My alter ego could attend these meetings, not me.

I was afraid of being judged. I was afraid of the pre-conceived ideas some of the support group women might have about "teachers" and "journalists." I didn't want any of them to think I was there to spy on them as parents, or report what they said to the newspaper. Or at least that's what I told myself.

And so I lived my lie. I figured I was doing everyone a

favor by assuming a separate Saturday morning identity. No one was getting hurt; it simply didn't matter. Or I thought it didn't matter, until the day I chaired that mid-winter meeting and reflected, for the first time, on what the willingness to become "honest" might mean to my ultimate recovery from compulsive overeating.

Of course, I had come clean with my best friend in the group when I'd asked her to help me with the program. We had spoken about my incessant need for anonymity, and she had agreed to keep my secret until I was ready to open that can of worms myself.

Later in the meeting, when it was my turn to share, I knew I had to confess. It was time to admit who I really was and take my lumps. I opened my mouth to speak, and totally choked. I made eye contact with my best food plan buddy. She nodded her support and handed me the tissues. The tears came fast and furious as I owned up to the deceit I had dished out for a full four and a half months.

I spoke without making eye contact with anyone. When I finished, I tentatively looked around the room. There was no criticism, no judgment, no blame, no finger pointing, and no "shame on you" showing on any face. No one even blinked.

I took my first deep and honest breath among my peers. I felt like I'd finally come home. Home to open arms of unconditional acceptance.

'Tis the season to gobble down the goodies

Statistics tell us the average American adult gains seven pounds between Thanksgiving and Christmas, and I had always prided myself on being "above average."

Now facing my first December committed to an honest-to-goodness bona fide healthy food plan, panic set in. What about those fabulous frosted sugar cookies with the red and green sprinkles? What about the bowls of red and green M&M candies I'd always kept on my desk? What about the endless platters of holiday snacks and goodies piled high on the staff room table?

What was this month-long celebration all about, if not about incomparable excess and overindulgence?

Each year for 15 years I had hosted a Christmas party in my home. I wasn't about to skip this annual tradition just because I was eating differently. Why should I deprive my friends the joy of getting together to sing carols around the piano and gorge themselves on a feast fit for kings and queens of all types?

My Christmas party was the highlight of my holidays. If I didn't have my seasonal soiree, I figured I might as well cross the entire month of December off the calendar and join some kind of pagan cult.

So I sent the handmade invitations and happily danced through the next two weeks in eager anticipation. I spent hundreds of dollars filling my freezer with a myriad of ready-made finger foods. I called it "Catering by Costco."

I whipped up seemingly endless batches of cashew clusters and mixed together all the hot spiced cider ingredients. And then I literally cried myself sick during the final preparations the night before. Terrific! Red, swollen eyes now accompanied my loudly growling stomach and rapidly deteriorating holiday mood.

What in the world had I been thinking? Most of the hors 'd oeuvres weighed in at 65 to 90 calories apiece, and there were more than a dozen bags of wings and poppers and taquitos and mini-egg rolls and two-bite cream puffs and every other type of heretofore forbidden food that had happened to catch my eye. There was more freakin' food in the house than I could legally eat on my food plan for months. *Many, many months!*

I finished putting post-it notes on all the platters covering the dining room table to remind me which food went where, and called David.

"Honey," he began, calming me immediately in his level-voiced, matter-of-fact way, "you will face many challenges in your new life. This is one of them. You have been faithfully following your plan for over two months. It's becoming ingrained as your new lifestyle. Defeat is not an option."

I called my best friend in the support group. "If it means this much to you, of course you can still have your party. Just make a decision not to sample as you set things up, and don't plan on having any leftovers."

No leftovers? But how could I guarantee that?

As I've said before, when you put a question out to the Universe, you've got to be willing to stop to listen, and then to be open and receptive to the answer.

I made a final trip to the grocery store the afternoon of the party. I bought extra ice and several boxes of heavy-duty plastic food storage bags, attractively decorated with little snowflakes. Designer freezer bags. Perfect.

A dozen times I read the nutrition information on all the ready-made hors d'oeuvres I'd purchased. I knew the exact caloric value of every single foodstuff I set out on the buffet table. Making a decision not to "graze" my way past the table during the party, I wrote out a list of what I could have for "dinner" when I finally decided it was time for me to eat. The list started with jumbo shrimp and cocktail sauce because I knew I could put a copious amount of those on my plate to help fill the space before getting to the much higher calorie items.

I loved playing the part of hostess. "The hostess with the mostest." A west coast Perle Mesta in the making. In my element, chatting, socializing, I flitted here and there from conversation to conversation while sipping on a diet soda. I refrained from putting *anything solid* into my mouth until almost 9 p.m.—perhaps not the best idea to postpone eating until that late in the evening, but I had a plan, and I was sticking to it. Then at 9 o'clock I calmly fixed myself a full plate of finger food. It was "dinnertime."

I sat on a folding chair next to an end table and tried to stop and savor each mouthful. My salivary glands worked overtime, making it difficult to eat slowly. I found myself resenting the "normal" eaters who nibbled at their food, often setting down their plates and wandering away without finishing. I couldn't imagine such behavior.

I polished off my one "legal" paper plate of food, considered licking the pattern off the paper, and my stomach told me I wanted *more*. Lots more…

This was the moment of truth. Although 12:30 a.m. New York time, I knew David stayed up late. I quietly walked down the hall, went into my bedroom, closed the door, and dialed his number. He answered on the first ring.

"How you doin', honey?" he immediately asked.

"I'm a little shaky," I admitted. I perched on the end of my bed, and sighed. "Talk to me."

And David patiently reminded me of all the reasons I had for choosing to save my life over having another plate, or two, or three, of food. "You have the power to get off the roller coaster," he said. "You've come too far to turn back now. You're not *really* hungry, you know, you're just falling back on your previous eating patterns."

I returned to the dining room and surveyed the scene. The party was beginning to wind down. I made an announcement that no one was leaving without a "doggie bag," and set out the decorated plastic food bags. "Please," I implored my friends as they gathered their coats, "help yourself! Take some home to your kids! Have a snack all ready for watching the football games tomorrow! Throw the food away when you get home if you want to, but *just take it!* I need you to help me get it out of here!"

Thankfully, most of them loaded up a bag or two. I felt blessed when it came time to do the post-party clean-up; there wasn't all that much food to put away. The relief that flooded through me was genuine. I bagged up individual "legal meals" and put them directly into the freezer.

A few women who sympathized with my struggles had been in attendance. "You did it," they whispered to me as they departed.

"No," I said honestly, "*We* did it. You, me and the Big Guy upstairs."

I wouldn't have been nearly so strong without knowing so many of my friends were right there beside me. It is only when you fail to plan that you plan to fail, and I had carefully planned for success. And the sweet taste of success contained no calories and no guilt.

I wrote down every single thing I'd eaten that day in my trusty food journal and was delighted to see the calorie count fall right in the middle of my target range. I had walked into the Valley of the Shadow of Death, and I had emerged *(with a lot of love and support from my friends and Higher Power)* victorious!

The next week was a little tough to navigate, what with plates of fudge and divinity and sugar cookies in the shape of stars and trees and bells everywhere I looked, but I stayed true to myself and my food plan. "Nothing tastes as good as thin feels," I told myself.

I called my support group buddy every day. "Together we can do what we could never do alone," she told me. "You don't have to eat like that anymore." I listened, and I began to believe in what she said.

Christmas 1999 fell on a Saturday. The support group met anyway. I passed out votive candles in holiday holders and thanked them for helping to light my path back from obesity. I thanked God for giving me the tools I needed to reclaim my life, and for putting a virtual parade of "Eskimos" in place for me every single day.

It was a wonderful Christmas, and I was on the verge of a wonderful new life.

Happy New Year 2000

Couples, couples everywhere. New Year's Eve must be the second loneliest night of the year for single folks, coming in a tight second behind Valentine's Day.

New Year's Eve to a single and perpetually dateless gal is about as much fun as having a root canal. New Year's Eve to a *morbidly obese*, single, and perpetually dateless gal is about as much fun as having a root canal without the benefit of novocaine.

But like it or not, December 31 rolled around and I looked frantically for a place to hide. I'm kind of funny about hiding, though. I don't like to be alone when I hide. I hide best when I'm in a crowd. Therefore, it was only natural for me to go out to a local bar and try to blend in with all the other single and dateless folks who are also looking to hide by being part of a group.

I did my best, but could only stomach it for an hour or so. I headed home shortly before 11 p.m., preferring *not* to be out there where some slobbering drunk might try to lay a kiss on me at midnight.

Or maybe I was just afraid that no one would *want* to kiss me as the clock struck 12. Who would want to kiss a female my size, other than some nearsighted blithering alcoholic, and probably a married one at that.

Nevertheless, as I watched the west coast's televised replay of the ball falling in Times Square, my tears also began to fall. Instead of welcoming a New Year and a fresh slate, I mourned the lost chances and missed opportunities of the previous decade. I cried buckets for every lonely New Year's Eve I'd ever spent, or ever would spend. I cried and cried and cried and cried, and then I stood in front of the open refrigerator door and cried some more.

I'd been following my food plan pretty religiously for almost three months, faithfully writing down everything I ate. That commitment alone had kept me "accountable" and doing well. And yet there I stood, "cooling the house down," as my mother would say, while searching for some forbidden foodstuff I somehow thought would help me numb the incredible and debilitating emotional pain.

I don't know who I thought would have filled my fridge with fattening favorites, perhaps the Bad Food Fairy or someone as equally insensitive, but I hungrily scanned each shelf with an eye to finding something, anything, I could grab and quickly stuff into my mouth before I had a chance to think about it. Old coping skills die hard, and I felt myself on the verge of backsliding yet again.

And then the phone rang. I glanced at the clock. 12:05 a.m. The fireworks display had not yet ended at the Seattle Center Space Needle. The echo of "Auld Lang Syne" still rang in my ears. I hit the "mute" button on the TV remote control and picked up the receiver.

"Happy New Year, honey!" said my angel's voice.

"David!" I exclaimed. "What on earth are you doing up? It's 3 a.m. in New York!"

"I didn't call to ask you the time in New York." He laughed. "I called because I wanted to be the first to wish you a Happy 2000—unless someone beat me to it."

"Your timing is impeccable," I replied, settling down in my recliner for a short but comfortable chat. "Thank God you called. Once again, you've saved me from myself."

"I'm here for you," he said. "I always will be. But you have to start giving yourself some of the credit for sticking with it, you know."

"I was so close to blowing it," I confessed. "Right now, this very minute, I knew I could screw it all up in a single heartbeat and go right back to where I was before I met you."

"No, no, you couldn't do that," David calmly replied. "It's a New Year, and you know you're on the right track. I have confidence in you. I only align myself with winners. The only reason for you to look over your shoulder is to see how far you've come."

I smiled. "Have I told you lately how much I appreciate your never-ending stream of platitudinal encouragement?"

"Yes," he answered without hesitation, and I could almost see the smirk on his face as he continued, "but don't quit telling me."

"I won't," I promised. "And David? I won't be overeating today, either."

"That's my girl," he said, and he bid me the sweetest and sveltest of dreams.

The telltale rocks

In January, 2000, I placed a wooden Lazy Susan on a forest green placemat on my dining room table and transformed it into a makeshift shrine. I needed a place to put my personal "items of inspiration and support," and creating a centerpiece seemed appropriate. Included were various greeting cards, pictures, scented candles, and the original purple and white polished marble "Hope" rock.

Each evening when I sat down to mindfully eat, observing these messages of love and caring helped me focus on the feelings rather than the food. "Nothing tastes as good as thin feels," I told myself night after night. "Easy does it. One day at a time. Trust the process. Stay in the present moment. You only have to refrain from compulsive overeating for one day. Just for today."

But I often felt anxious and disappointed at how slowly I progressed. Sometimes I felt resentful and even angry I was working so hard and yet my weight wasn't disappearing nearly fast enough to suit me. I wrestled my roiling emotions daily and I frequently whined by telephone to David and my special support buddy that I'd better start seeing more dramatic results if there was going to be any hope of me sticking to my program.

"Look how far you've come," David told me again and again and again and again. "Your new way of eating is becoming a way of life. Don't give up now."

"It's not about the numbers," said my support friend. "It's about becoming healthier emotionally and spiritually as well as physically."

I listened to them with half an ear. I heard them, but I didn't take their words completely into heart. I wanted (*and felt I needed*) the tangible "proof" all this trouble was worth it. I wanted to have the weight leave me like shucking off an old winter coat. I wanted a total caterpillar to butterfly metamorphosis, and I wanted it *yesterday.*

Late in the month, one of the women in my Saturday support group came to the meeting bearing gifts. Like a mysterious sorceress, she shook and rattled the contents of a brown paper bag in front of each of us. "Reach inside," she said with a mischievous grin, "and find out what gifts the Universe is giving you today."

Around the group she went, having each of us select, without looking, two acrylic "crafters' pebbles." These pebbles were a little larger than a dime, flat on the bottom and rounded on the top. They were the type used in vases, aquariums, to decorate picture frames, lampshades, and lots of other "artsy" projects.

These particular pebbles had once been clear colored glass, but the woman, being an artsy type herself, had altered them. Each one now had a word of encouragement glued to the bottom so we could read the message by peering right through the pebble. She'd also added a sprinkle of glitter. No two pebbles bore the same message.

Drawing out my two miniature pseudo-rocks, I felt a lot like I do when opening a fortune cookie. There was a rush of eager anticipation as I pondered what the future might hold. But with this particular form of prognostication, there were no forbidden cookie calories attached.

I reached inside the bag, withdrew my prize, and paused before looking at the pebbles. The other women's eyes were all upon me as I finally took a deep breath and read the messages aloud. "Patience" and "Gratitude."

There was a moment of utter silence. Then everyone in the room joined me as I totally cracked up laughing. It was as if a divine 2 by 4 had struck me square between the eyes.

Bingo! We have a winner!

I had gotten the two words I needed most. The Universe had heard my fervent prayers for help and once again miraculously answered them in an unmistakable way. God had given me a sign so big even I couldn't miss it.

Back home, I added the pebbles to my ever-growing shrine-in-progress. I placed them right beside "Hope" for my continued contemplation. Hope, Patience, and Gratitude—three very important words I'd be a fool not to hang onto.

In glorious black and white

Following a well-balanced food plan will eventually result in weight loss. But as everyone knows, at least intellectually, exercise is the key to burning maximum calories and taking the pounds off just a little bit faster.

Exercise and I were no strangers to each other. I had participated in a variety of organized sports throughout high school. And even after an absence of many years, my muscle memory was still intact.

I wrote "Get more exercise" on my list of New Year's resolutions the first of every January. And every year I made a good stab at sticking to it by setting up a daily walking schedule. Some years I was still walking regularly into late February or the first few weeks of March.

Walking is relatively low-impact and takes no special equipment other than a good pair of tennis shoes. But walking has its drawbacks. When I walked along the road near my home, I took my life into my hands.

The shoulder of the road is far too narrow for anyone to walk safely. Teen-agers in passing cars often threw things at me as I strode along. It was hurtful and humiliating. Pop cans, milkshakes, cigarette butts and apple cores were hurled in my direction. And I admit, at my size I made a pretty easy target.

Walking on the beach was difficult as well. The soft sand failed to support my girth and my knees were not sturdy enough to go very far. I could walk on the half-mile boardwalk, and I often did, but that meant I had to drive into town to get there. It wasn't always convenient for me to drop everything to do that. I guess I just wasn't willing to go to any lengths to get the exercise I knew I needed.

The swimming pool, however, was much closer to my home. They were open a couple evenings a week, and there was even a little old ladies' water aerobics class available. It sounded like the answer to another of my prayers.

Only one thing held me back. I needed a swimsuit. A *very large* swimsuit. And there wasn't anyplace nearby which sold swimsuits in the middle of the winter, much less *very large* swimsuits.

So I scoured the specialty catalogs and finally found a swimsuit I felt would cover enough of me so going to the pool wouldn't cause me to suffer too much shame. I put a rush on the order and it arrived two days later. The day it came happened to be a day the evening exercise class met.

At 5:45 I pulled on my swimsuit and took a good look in the mirror. I turned this way and that. The suit was black and white, and while it covered what it needed to cover, it also accentuated the three or four rolls of fat cascading down my belly, back, and butt. I thought I looked like a giant Emperor penguin, or maybe Shamu the killer whale.

I wore my suit under my bathrobe for the drive to the pool so I wouldn't have to change in front of anyone when I got there. I shucked out of my robe in the dressing room and descended the steps into the water quicker than I thought I could move. Once in the water, I maneuvered until I was about chin deep to do the exercises. I didn't want anyone looking at me, or feeling sorry for me. I felt sorry enough for myself.

I must say I gave it my best shot. But there was no way on God's green earth I could even pretend to be keeping up with the instructor. The little old ladies were stirring up a real froth and I was in constant danger of being swamped.

I tried doing the exercises at half speed, but that didn't help much. I got totally out of breath and working up one heck of a sweat while standing in a *swimming pool!*

Discouraged but not defeated, I returned to the class a second time. And a third. And a fourth. And soon I became one of the die-hard few that never missed a session. I have no fathomable idea what got me to go back time after time, unless, once again, there was a Higher Power at work on my behalf. It must have been God who gave me the courage to continue—the courage to change the things I can, and the willingness to do so.

After several months, I had modified the exercises and did my own thing in the deep water by myself. I could still hear and enjoy the music, and I was still moving, and I knew moving, however minimal, had to be better than being at home sitting, or lying, on the couch.

After a little more than three months, a funny thing happened. I was doing a series of "push-ups" against the side of the pool when both my breasts suddenly popped out of my swimsuit. No one was exercising near me, so I just stopped and pushed them back inside the foam cups. A few minutes later they popped out a second time.

I laughed hysterically and swallowed a lot of pool water. I started choking and sputtering. The lifeguard walked rapidly around to my end of the pool.

"Are you okay?"

"I'm fine," I told her truthfully. "I'm better than fine. I think, though, that it's about time I got a new swimsuit."

I didn't bother to explain, and the next week I showed up in a hot fuchsia pink flowered and softly skirted number.

"You've lost weight," the lifeguard immediately said.

"Yes I have," I replied. "And I decided it was time to add a little color to my life. I don't want to be mistaken for a celebrity killer whale any longer."

"A celebrity killer whale?"

"That's right," I said, filling her in on the story. Then I pointed to first one breast and then the other. "Meet 'Free' — and 'Willy'."

CHAPTER IV:
ONE HUNDRED POUNDS DOWN

Crosses to bear

Mid-March of 2000, I read about a gathering of other compulsive overeaters who were meeting at a coastal retreat center a couple hours south of where I live. I'd been feeling I needed some kind of intense booster shot to help me stick with my program, and the price for the weekend (*including all food!*) was very reasonable.

I paid my conference fee and arrived on the designated Friday night in plenty of time to look the place over in drizzling daylight. It was laid out like any other camp of this type. Clusters of cabins and dormitory-like buildings surrounded a main hall and cafeteria.

There were lots of other women, and even a few men, wandering here and there as I was, acclimating themselves to the facility.

My assigned dorm room sported bunk beds with thin plastic-covered mattresses that promised unrelenting squeaks whenever a person turned over.

I had borrowed two sleeping bags to zip together so I wouldn't feel the tight confinement of an unforgiving ace-bandage cocoon all night, but I worried I'd never be able to sleep in such close quarters with five other women.

I've always preferred the privacy of having my own

room, and considered checking into a nearby motel, but I decided to reserve judgment and give it one night.

Dinner was "family style," and I felt a sudden wave of uncertainty and disorientation passing around the bowls and platters. I didn't know if what we had on the table was all we were getting to eat, or if the serving pieces would be refilled if we ran short at our table set for eight.

I was worried about getting enough to eat, yes, but also worried everyone there was probably more under control in the food department than me. For the past six months I had avoided buffet lines and potluck dinners.

Having the food right there, but having others with similar issues surrounding food also right there, put me in a state of terrible tension. I was sure they were all members of the secret "food police" and bells and buzzers and sirens would go off if I put more on my plate than allowed.

My throat constricted and a sense of panic prevailed. I felt like bolting from the room and not stopping till I was safe and sound at a nice, predictable, drive-thru window. It's hard to explain why I was so distressed over eating in front of other eaters. I just hoped I could blend in.

Thankfully, some of my dining companions had attended this type of weekend retreat before and I followed their lead. I still felt a little hungry after most of the others had finished their meals, and there was still food on the table. Previously, I would have picked at the "leftovers" and cleaned up every dish not already empty.

I could see my anxious reflection in the eyes of a few women at the table. I wasn't alone in my thoughts, and somehow there was security in knowing that. I silently added up my calories, decided that it wasn't actually hunger I was experiencing, and left the table with food still within my reach. A minor miracle.

I went back to the dorm room to get my notebook and pen before the keynote speaker began. Sitting on the edge of the lower bunk bed, I debated again whether this whole retreat thing was such a good idea. I thought about the outdoor camp I'd attended in sixth grade, and how all the girls had put their heads together to share their smuggled candy, chips, and other snacks.

I was curious if any of the suitcases today contained such "forbidden" treats. I already knew there was a game room complete with several junk food vending machines in the basement of the meeting hall just a few short yards away. And I knew I had plenty of coins in my purse.

Before I let that thought progress any further, however, I went to the communal bathroom to splash some cold water on my face.

A very attractive woman in her 40s entered the bathroom. My first thought was to wonder what in the world *she* was doing at this conference; she was absolutely gorgeous! What I wouldn't have given to look like she did!

My second thought was maybe she had been a few pounds heavier at some point and was now maintaining her goal weight. In that case, she could certainly be an inspiration to me. But when her eyes met mine, she looked like the metaphorical deer caught in the headlights. Or maybe in our case, she was a kid caught with her hand in the cookie jar. A long moment passed.

"I didn't know anyone else would be in here," she said.

I was a bit taken aback. There were a half dozen stalls with doors, a wall of mirrors behind several sinks, and even a few private showers in the room. It wasn't like she had to stand in line to use the facilities. But something in my gut told me to tread gently. "Would you like me to leave?"

She dropped her eyes and took a deep breath. Another

long moment crawled by. "I'm bulimic," she said softly.

It took me a minute to grasp what she was getting at. "Would you like me to leave?" I asked again.

She shook her head. "What I'd *like* is to be able to enjoy eating a nice healthy meal like we just finished and not find it necessary to immediately purge. What I'd *like* is to be able to eat like a normal person and not be afraid I was gaining 10 pounds every time I swallowed a pitifully small quantity of food."

I'd never knowingly met a bulimic before. "Do you force yourself to throw up after *every* meal?" I asked incredulously.

She sighed. "I started purging years ago whenever I ate a whole box of chocolate cupcakes or a dozen candy bars or a ton of something I knew wasn't good for me. Laxatives didn't work fast enough. I needed to get the offending junk out of me before my body absorbed any of the calories. I'm actually a compulsive eater who controls her weight by sticking her finger down her throat."

I sat down on the bench next to the row of shower stalls and listened attentively while she told me her story. I just listened. I didn't judge, counsel, interrupt, or offer advice.

When she finished speaking, we shared a few private minutes of quiet reflection. Then I said, "Whenever I meet someone, they can quickly *see* that I have an eating disorder. It's obvious just by looking at me. But you—you look so—'normal'…"

She smiled. "We all have our crosses to bear."

I smiled back. "So do you want me to leave now, or do you want to go with me to the evening speaker session?"

"We're only as sick as our secrets," she replied, "and my eating disorder is not a secret anymore."

We laughed and cried together as we listened to our

stories being told again and again by not only the keynote speaker, but by every man and woman who got up to share. Compulsive eaters, sneak eaters, bulimics, anorexics, extremist exercisers, laxative addicts—we all had the very same stories, and it was wildly comforting to know that we were not nuts, and we were most certainly not alone.

My dis-ease had caused me to isolate at home for many years. Here in the midst of these courageously recovering food addicts, I felt a definite sense of belonging—and hope.

What does "under 300" feel like?

March 27, 2000: A day that will live in infamy. On March 27, 2000, I saw something I hadn't seen on a scale in over a decade. I saw a "two" as the first digit of my weight. I had spent the entire decade of the 90s above 300 pounds, and on this glorious day in March, just nine months and one day after making the decision (*with the not-so-gentle prodding of my counselor*) to commit to saving my life, I had lost 97 pounds, and now weighed "just" 299.

Absolutely unbelievable. Only in my extremely fertile imagination had I dared to hope I would *ever* be under 300 pounds again in this lifetime. When I saw the needle on the scale register a good hair's breadth below the double zeros, I laughed, I cried, and I wanted to go out and celebrate—with food.

No kidding. As odd as it may sound, the thing I most wanted to do to commemorate this historic event was to go out and enjoy a very nice dinner. Splurge a little. Pamper myself. Indulge. After all, I certainly deserved it.

Fortunately, before I fell headlong into the obvious trap I was setting, I shared my success with my support group study-buddy.

"Congratulations!" she exclaimed. "And you know, of course, this is a potentially dangerous moment for relapse."

Relapse? Whatever was she talking about? I had no intention of gaining back any *weight*, I just wanted to go out for one really good meal. Celebrating with food was something I had learned very early in life, and I had no alternative plans yet in place.

On the phone with my support friend, we talked about the dangers inherent in thinking the worst was over. For a compulsive eater, *every day* is the worst day. Compulsive behavior never takes a holiday; it never cuts us any slack. Every day we either move forward or fall backward. The choice to eat sanely must be made anew each day.

"If you rest on your laurels, your laurels will get bigger." I remembered that slogan from one of our meetings. My friend chimed in with an entire string of trite, but nevertheless appropriate, sayings and slogans.

As we chatted, my gaze fell on a clipping taped to the wall beside my computer. Regrettably, I had not included the proper attribution to this motivating paragraph. I have no recollection on my frame of mind at the time I taped it there, but I know it had nothing to do with my food obsession. More likely, I put the clipping there to encourage me to continue my fledgling freelance writing.

These words of inspiration had been in front of me for 12 full years, but as I read them again, they took on a whole new meaning:

"Something in human nature causes us to start slacking off at our moment of greatest accomplishment. As you become successful, you will need a great deal of self-discipline not to lose your sense of balance, humility, and commitment."

I got goose bumps. That quote has been there since long before I ever even *thought* of following a food plan. It had been there, waiting for me for over a decade, quietly, constantly, lurking in the background. All I had to do was read it with new eyes to see the wisdom as it pertained to my continued recovery from compulsive eating.

Instead of going out to dinner, I made a list of rewards. Calorie-free rewards. Rewards like earrings, lottery tickets, a make-up makeover, a new outfit, a movie date with myself in a theater where now I thought I just might be able to squeeze myself into the seat, a new Ricky Martin CD to play in the car, and perhaps a trip to Las Vegas.

Las Vegas! Now there was an idea aptly fit for the truly obsessive/compulsive person! One-armed bandits! Endless buffets! All night entertainment!

Naturally, I booked my celebratory trip to the country of countless land mines the very next day.

Flying solo: The view from the back of the plane

My stomach wrenched as I stood in line to get my boarding pass for the plane to Las Vegas. What if I didn't fit into the seat? What if I needed a seatbelt extender? What if the people sitting next to me complained I oozed over into their personal space?

When my turn came at the counter, I asked if there were any empty rows left. The woman dumbly stared at me for a moment, then checked the computer. "There's no one yet assigned to the back three rows," she said. "Back by the bathroom." She lowered her voice. "They aren't very good seats—no one ever requests to sit there."

"Will I get to Las Vegas at the same time as everyone

else?" I asked.

She again looked at me quizzically, and then replied deadpan, "You'll actually arrive ahead of the rest of them. The back of the plane touches down first."

"Suits me just fine," I said, as she marked the seat assignment on my boarding pass with a felt-tipped pen.

I stowed my carry-on overhead and put all the arm rests in the row up and out of the way before I settled into the middle seat of three. I exhaled deeply and slid the seatbelt buckle all the way to the end before attempting to fasten it around me. I sucked in my stomach for all I was worth and swung my arm over my belly.

The strap snapped into place. I took a breath. So far, so good. Then, to my amazement, I discovered I could actually adjust the belt a teensy-weensy bit snugger. I felt a surprising surge of confidence as I released the latch to lower the tray table in front of me.

My confidence was short-lived. The tray table's progress was arrested by my still-protruding stomach and stopped quite a bit short of lying flat. I quickly put the tray back up; the familiar rush of embarrassment flushed my cheeks, and I was thankful no one had witnessed what I considered an epic fail.

Fortunately, the only food served during the flight was a bag of peanuts, which I easily declined, and a diet soft drink, which I held in my hand until I finished drinking it. I suppose I could have put down the tray on the adjoining seatback, but I didn't want to draw attention to my plight.

I departed the plane in Las Vegas without incident, located a shuttle to transport me to my hotel, and began absorbing the ambience of glowing neon.

By the time I reached my destination, my initial joy at being able to fit into an airline seat had returned. I couldn't wait to get checked in at the hotel and start checking out all the sights and sounds surrounded me. The new and improved me. The less than 300 pound me.

I had arrived!

Sin City

I had four nights and almost five whole days in Las Vegas to play to my heart's content. I planned to begin and end each day with a swim in the hotel pool. That was the plan. So after a quick perusal of my room, I pulled on my swimsuit and robe, grabbed a towel, and took the elevator to the bottom floor.

Here I was, a two hundred ninety-something pound woman frothing around in a Las Vegas swimming pool. Las Vegas: Home of the five-foot, ten-inch, size-six show girls. I struggled valiantly not to feel shame over my size. Let them stare! I would never see these people again! Well, I couldn't actually *see* them now, because I'm nearsighted and I swim with my glasses off.

But back in my room, my bravado collapsed. The interior decorator of this hotel, in an apparent effort to give the room more light and a greater sense of space, had paneled two abutting walls with bamboo-latticed mirrors. This motif extended to the ceiling as well.

After removing my swimsuit, I sat naked on the bed, towel-drying my hair. I put my glasses on, looked up, and contemplated my reflection. The abundant rolls of my pale flesh, viewed from above, totally appalled me. Viewed from any angle, my fat was not pretty, but from this vantage point, three competing impressions immediately battled for prominence in my conscious mind.

One: I looked like the animated Michelin Tire Man from the television commercials, my body composed of one white spare tire piled rakishly upon another.

Two: I looked like a naked, over-kneaded and distinctly lumpy Pillsbury Doughboy wannabe.

Three: I looked like a swirled Tastee-Freeze ice cream cone slowly melting into a mushy puddle of soft-serve.

These graphic images conspired to ruin my entire trip. I had lost approximately 100 pounds and was "on vacation" to celebrate that accomplishment. Yet here I sat, completely immersed in self-loathing. I had released *one hundred freaking pounds*, and it still wasn't enough. I felt miserable. No matter how much I lost, it might not ever be enough.

I allowed myself a good cry. Then, puffy eyes and all, I somehow managed to shake it off and get dressed, gather what was left of my composure, and head for the casino. The noise, the lights, the bells, buzzers, whistles and eclectic assortment of people would surely distract me from my self-deprecating thoughts.

Six hours and several hundred dollars later, I went looking for less expensive distractions. I got tickets for several shows, and had my first-ever professional manicure. And then, finally succumbing to the growing rumble in my stomach, I went looking for food. Healthy food.

Buffets, however, are not healthy in any way, shape or form. I *knew* that, but I got into line for one anyway. And as I stood there, inching my way forward, I had time to observe the abundance of choices soon to be available at my sole discretion. I felt a familiar tightening in my throat. My respiration became shallow. I got clammy all over. My knees threatened to discontinue supporting me and I was seriously afraid I might faint.

I stepped out of line and took refuge on a nearby stool

to gather my wits. My extreme physical reaction, I rationalized, must be the result of not having eaten all day. It was just low blood sugar. I'd be fine in a minute. I just needed to sit and think this through. I'd be damned if I was going to throw away my entire food plan all because the sign above the cash register said "All you can eat."

A casino attendant approached me. "Do you need help with this machine?" he asked.

Until then I hadn't even looked to see what type of machine my security stool was bellied up to. I swiveled around and came face to face with an electronic device I had not encountered while living in a small coastal town.

"What is this?" I asked the attendant. "Where am I?"

He laughed. "It's called an Internet Cafe," he replied. "You put cash or credit card into the appropriate slot and you buy minutes so you can surf the 'net or check your email. Want me to show you how?"

Through the fog of my confusion, a light dawned. My Higher Power had sent me yet another demonstration of Divine Intervention. This man was another Eskimo and dinner could wait a few more minutes.

"Yes, please," I said with a smile. "I think I'm in email withdrawal."

And with a few simple mouse clicks, I called up my email and read what I already knew would be waiting for me—several messages of love and support from my compulsive eating sisters back home.

I quickly typed out a reply to one of them, pressed "send," and took a deep breath. I knew I was not alone as I walked past the buffet and found a small deli where I bought a mayonnaise-free hoagie sandwich and a plate of assorted fruit. God was indeed good. As I added up my calories, I remembered to count my blessings, too.

After dinner I took a short walk. The noises of the city were amazing. I enjoyed the experience, so different than walking on my isolated home beach. Soon I was inextricably drawn to the roller coaster in front of the New York, New York, casino.

I used to love roller coasters. I used to love the thrill, the rush, the implied danger. But now I watched passively as others shrieked and screamed and I coveted their release of pumped-up adrenalin.

But there was no point in trying to fool myself. I knew I couldn't safely fit into the seat for the ride. And even if I did manage to squeeze myself in, the harness and the lap bar didn't have a prayer of securing a person my size. My experience with the tray table on the plane kept me from becoming delusional. "Not this time," I told myself. "But next time, I promise."

I walked away with a deep sense of sadness, but also a renewed sense of determination. I desperately wanted to fit into the seat of that amusement ride. I will ride that roller coaster, I vowed to myself, "someday soon."

My entire time in Vegas was laced with such dichotomies. One moment I was up, and positive, and full of energy and commitment, and the next I was plummeting into the emotional abyss, certain I didn't have a snowball's chance in hell of achieving my goals.

The entire vacation was bittersweet—like my favorite chocolate—but I had voluntarily walked into this land of assorted decadence, and I had triumphed. I came home ready, willing, and able to tackle the next 100 pounds.

Facing down the Department of Drivers' Licensing

As happens every year about this time, my birthday arrived the first week of June, 2000. I was 46 years old and weighed 272 pounds. I noted this event with some quiet introspection. Thirty years earlier, in my junior year of high school, I'd been 16 years old and weighed 145 pounds. My participant number at the state track meet that season had been #272. I still had the placard.

What goes around, comes around, I sadly mused.

The numbers on the scale were slowly and surely decreasing, but instead of seeing how far I'd come, I was obsessing about how far I had yet to go. The previous year I had weighed 124 pounds heavier. What I had accomplished in the past year was truly amazing! I had released an average of just over 10 pounds a month for a full year! And yet I was hit daily by reminders I was far from fitting my weight on the chart proclaiming the insurance norms.

Another gruesome reminder of my yet-to-be-realized goal was the reality check I got when I went to get my driver's license renewed.

After waiting for over two hours, an unheard of amount of time in our small rural community, I was finally motioned to the desk. I smiled and told the man I could wait another few minutes if he needed to take a break or anything. He returned my smile, but said he was fine.

With my glasses on, I pressed my forehead against the monitor and easily read the lowest line on the eye chart. Then the clerk asked me if I still wanted to maintain my motorcycle endorsement. I assured him I did. He asked if I still wanted to be an organ donor. Again I answered affirmatively.

My home had been assigned a more specific address

since I'd last renewed my license, so instead of the simple route and mail box number, I dictated my new house numbers while he took the time to type them into the computer data bank.

He sighed and scanned the rest of my expiring card. I confirmed my name remained unchanged. He read aloud as he entered hair color, eye color, and "corrective lenses."

He paused. All too well, I knew the next section contained my height and weight. I held my breath, wondering how I would answer his next inquiry. I thought I could admit to maybe 220 or 240, but whatever number I told him now would remain on my license for at least the next 4 years, and I balked at the thought of that admission staying with me for so long.

"Is there anything else on your license you'd like to change?" he asked, with another audible sigh. The man was a true diplomat. But he was obviously not aware of my innate ability to turn his leading question into a game of simple semantics.

I hesitated. I thought very carefully about the phrasing of his question. Very, very, *very* carefully. After what must have been a month or better, I looked him square in the eye and confidently replied, "No, sir. There is nothing else on my driver's license that I would like you to change."

He held my gaze. Then he looked at the clock. It was 5:35. The office had officially closed at 5 p.m. I was his last customer of the day. He looked again at my license. He typed a few more strokes into the computer and then turned back to me. He patiently smiled again as he said, "Please step up to the green line and look straight into the camera."

I did as told. My license printed out in a matter of moments, I handed the nice man my check, and I was out the door and on my way.

I walked down the block and got into my car before I dared to look at the new card in my hand. In the space where my weight was recorded it said exactly what it had said when I first got it 30 years previous at age 16. It said I weighed 145 pounds.

The smile in my driver's license picture is absolutely priceless.

No greater gift

Every year I use my birthday to reflect not only on the passing of another milestone, but to write my New Year's Resolutions. That's right—resolutions. While others may choose to indulge in this activity on January 1st, I prefer to review the year and list my goals according to my birth calendar. It is, after all, the start of my very own New Year.

In 2000, I kept the list fairly simple: Continue with my food and exercise plan, go horseback riding on the beach, catch a couple "legal-sized" sturgeon, test drive a Corvette, fall in love, and have sex.

Continuing with my food and exercise plan was a given, and it topped my list because it was, and forever would be, the most important thing in my life.

I hadn't ridden a horse since I was 15 or 16, and my darling niece was now 10 years old and totally into the horseback riding on the beach thing. And I desperately wanted to be able to go with her.

Two of my dear friends had a boat, and had invited me to go fishing with them, so I was already half way to my sturgeon-catching goal.

Since my high school graduation in 1972, I had wanted

to drive a Corvette. I had harbored this dream for 28 years, and it was time to follow through. I didn't think I could comfortably fit into anything approximating a sports car at my current size, but as soon as I thought I was able, finding one to test drive was a done deal.

That left falling in love and having sex. At the time I wrote my list, it had been years since I'd felt like any kind of sexual being. I even considered I perhaps I had "outgrown" wanting to feel sexy and desirable. Perhaps the estrogen lurking in the fat had taken away my libido. If the truth be told, it had been about a decade since I'd gotten naked and horizontal with anyone. I wasn't just hormonally challenged—I was hormonally comatose.

At the time I wrote my list, I thought falling in love and having sex went hand in hand. Normally, one would assume falling in love immediately preceded sex. But not necessarily. The universal Divine Mind is always listening, and everything happens in its own time.

Just three days after I wrote my birthday resolutions, I got a call from a very good longtime friend who told me he was in town for a short visit and wondered if we could get together to catch up on old times.

Well, in the old times, we had never been intimate, and in the old times we had never shared more than a hug and a quick kiss hello or goodbye. And besides, I was 272 pounds for crying out loud, and a long ways from applying for the role of fem fatale, so I was extremely confident there was no way we'd be "going there" now.

But like I said, the universal Divine Mind often has other ideas.

After a few minutes of polite conversation, my longtime platonic friend put his arm around me and pulled me tight against him. His kiss was much more than a friendly greeting, and I felt myself swoon. To my knowledge, I had never actually swooned before, but I instantly knew what was happening.

Hand in hand, we walked down the hall to my bedroom, and he insisted on undressing me himself, right then and there, in full daylight and with no place for me to hide. I flushed scarlet and tried to protest, but he shook his head and told me to hush.

We spent the entire afternoon enjoying the full pleasure of each other's company. For the first time in too many years to count, I felt treasured, cherished, appreciated, and very sexually aroused. My libido, I discovered, was very much alive and well.

As the afternoon wound to a close, I modestly reached down to pull the sheet up over me. My friend gently stopped my hand and softly asked me if I were cold.

"No…" I replied. "I— I just want to pull the sheet up."

"Why?" he challenged.

"You know why," I answered. The lump in my throat felt like a brick. I turned my head away.

"Oh, honey." He pulled me tightly into his arms again, but I still couldn't meet his eyes.

He lightly kissed my forehead, then my nose, then a quick kiss on the lips. "Your body is just fine," he said. "You don't need to hide it from me or anyone else. You're a very sexy woman no matter what your size. Don't you understand that?"

I started to cry.

"What's all this?" he asked, taking my face in his hands and wiping his thumbs softly across my cheeks to brush away the tears.

I tried to put my feelings into words, but everything I opened my mouth to say seemed extremely inadequate.

Finally I managed to whisper, "Thank you."

I'd never had a birthday present better than the warm glow that comes with unconditional size acceptance.

What price, commercial recovery centers?

In mid-June, 2000, my counselor again suggested I attend an inpatient program. She felt that since I had gotten under 300 pounds I had lost a little of the sense of urgency to my recovery, and complacency was the enemy.

I thought we'd been through all this the previous summer. I had no intention of going away to a treatment center and then coming home to the same old mindset, the same old "let's celebrate with food" friends, the same old job challenges, and so forth. I could not see what good it would do to go away for a month and come home to the previous status quo.

How much weight could a person lose in 30 days? It wasn't like I could disappear from my home and responsibilities and come home slim and trim a couple weeks later. If that were the case, I'd have already gone.

I am a very stubborn woman, but my counselor and I now had almost a year invested together, and well aware of the fact I was paying to listen to her advice.

Listening to her advice, however, did not necessarily mean I would take it. Nevertheless, not wanting to waste my counseling money, I decided to check into the logistics of going to an overeating recovery center, just to humor her, if nothing else.

On the Internet, I got one heck of a rude awakening. While bulimia and anorexia are considered eating disorders, I could find very little information on treatment centers offering help for the compulsive overeater. Apparently, compulsive overeating was not an actual disease in the minds of most insurance companies, mine included, and therefore a treatment center didn't qualify as a viable medical condition.

After searching for hours, I found only two centers where my specific problem was even addressed. I explored the multi-page information on those sites, acutely aware of a lack of costs listed. If a restaurant doesn't post its prices on the menu, one just knows it's going to be expensive.

I dialed the 1-800 number for a center in California. A very cordial woman answered the phone and danced all around my questions about money while she inquired as to my type of insurance and my current level of commitment and gave me the total third degree about my general health.

Finally, after much insistence on my part, she lowered the monetary boom. "Our 30-day program for compulsive overeaters is available for $1400 a day," she said as matter-of-factly as if she were telling me the price of a McDonald's Happy Meal.

"I'm sorry, I must not have heard you correctly. Did you say $1400 *a day?*"

"That is correct," she replied, still without a trace of embarrassment. "If you'll check out our website calendar, you'll see that what we offer is 24-hour support and assistance in every facet of weight loss. If you want to get well and stay well, the money is irrelevant."

Maybe it was irrelevant *to her*, but as for me, I was stunned. Speechless. Totally overwhelmed. My math skills are very good, and I didn't need a calculator to multiply $1400 times 30 days and come up with a whopping $42,000 for the treatment package, and that wasn't even including the airfare to get there! *Forty-two thousand dollars!*

"I just checked on your insurance," she continued as if I were still paying attention and had not succumbed to incapacitating shock, "and it pays a lifetime $20,000 for this type of program. You can contact them yourself, or we can do that for you when we officially sign you up. We have openings in two weeks, if that's convenient to your schedule. We accept VISA and MasterCard."

My brain turned to mush. I couldn't even think of a snappy comeback. Somehow I managed to mumble, "I'll have to think some more about this," before I hung up.

It suddenly occurred to me I couldn't *afford* any other plan than the one I had been working on my own for the past year. I wasn't wealthy enough to check myself in, even if I wanted to. And just as suddenly, I found myself *resenting* not being able to get the professional help I needed. I was angry at the entire health care system, and mad at the world for making my disease nothing more than a "for profit" business opportunity.

Fortunately for me, when I get mad, I take action.

Do-it-yourself retreat

Where there's a will, there's a way, and I suddenly had an abundance of will. How dare they make me feel I couldn't afford to go to their dumb old retreat center! I'll show them, I vowed, and went back online to re-examine the elements of their proposed program.

I located the sample weekly calendar for the institute and wrote down all the classes, sessions, and opportunities available. Among other things, they offered individual counseling, small group counseling, larger support meetings, nutrition classes, a variety of exercise classes, and required readings along with written homework.

My teacher training kicked right in; my lesson plan was going to be a virtual low-fat, calorie-free, piece of cake.

But first I needed a safe haven for my self-created hiatus. After considering my options, I picked up the phone and called my friend Steve, in Hailey, Idaho. "Can I come hang out at your place for a week or two?" I asked.

In less than a heartbeat, he answered affirmatively. "I'll be working every day," he said, "but you're welcome to come and stay as long as you wish."

I briefly outlined my idea, and asked him to do a little local research for me, to which he again readily agreed.

On previous trips east, I had become familiar with every type of food available at every freeway exit between my house and Steve's—every fast-food fix at every drive-thru window. It took a lot of determination and plenty of fortitude for me to keep on driving by all those "comfort stations," even when I knew in my heart I didn't really *need* any gas or a bathroom break.

By the time I arrived at his home a few days later, Steve had done his homework. He handed me a list of all kinds of support groups in the area, along with the times and days and locations where they met. He also had the schedule for the local swimming pool and gave me information on water aerobics classes and introductory yoga.

As he helped me carry box after box of magazines, books, cassettes and video tapes in from the car, Steve must have wondered if I was moving in permanently. But I was a woman on a mission, and I was determined to make the most out of my do-it-yourself retreat experience.

I stayed at Steve's place for 11 days. In that time I read dozens of fitness, nutrition, and cooking light magazines. I listened to inspirational cassette tapes from others who had

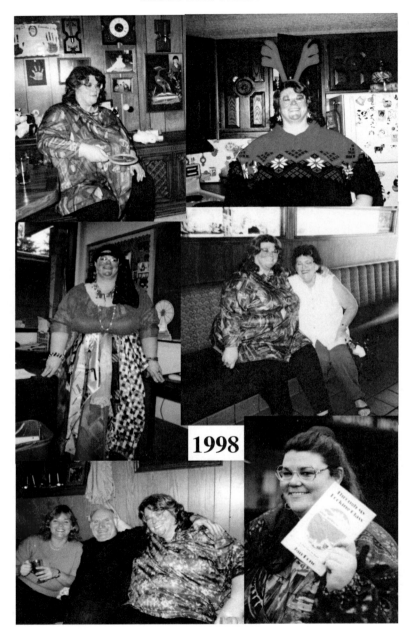

1998

138

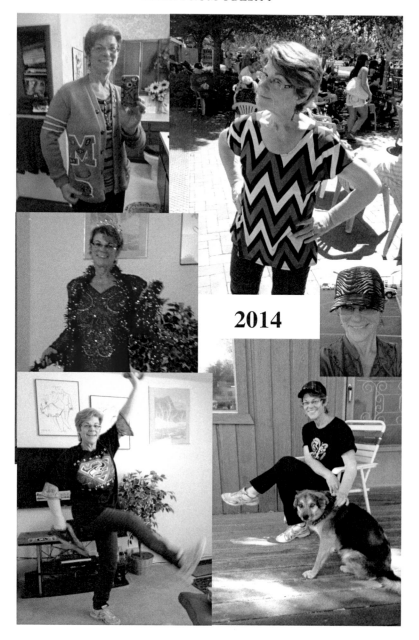

2014

lost weight, and I gleaned important tidbits on how they now maintained a healthier lifestyle. I went to water aerobics class every morning, and exercised while watching a videotape every afternoon. In the evenings, Steve and I often went for a walk together.

I did all the cooking while I was there. That was the least I could do for my rent-free haven in Hailey. Steve was following a low carbohydrate diet at the time, and I incorporated that into my menu planning while I tried out many of the new recipes I found during my afternoon magazine reading time.

I wrote copiously in my journal, and attended every support group meeting within a 20-mile radius, whether I had that particular addiction or not. I settled my butt into a meeting chair three times a day—at 7 a.m., noon, and 7 p.m. I went to meetings not only in Hailey, but also in the neighboring towns of Bellevue and Ketchum.

At one meeting in Ketchum, I met a man from the east coast who had lost over 100 pounds and had kept it off for 18 years already. I asked him if it was really necessary for him to continue attending the support groups, to which he immediately replied, "If you rest on your laurels, your laurels will get bigger." I smiled and nodded my familiarity with his advice; I'd heard that saying once or twice before.

He gave me the email address of an online group of people who had all lost over 100 pounds. Shocked that such a group existed, it was as if a new door had suddenly opened and I quickly stepped through it.

I'd felt so isolated before, having never met anyone locally who had had success doing what I was doing. Now I knew I wasn't alone; I wasn't terminally unique! There were people just like me somewhere out there after all!

It was as if I were coming home to the friendship and

acceptance I'd been craving all along. Intellectually, I had known we are always so much stronger when we surround ourselves with others in a similar situation, but in reality, I had not known where or how to connect with others with very similar challenges.

What a demonstration of Divine Intervention for a woman from the very edge of the west coast to connect with a man from clear across the country in a remote little town in central Idaho who would be able to give her all the answers she'd been seeking! God, once again, had placed an Eskimo in my path at a critical juncture in my coming to terms with my disease.

And what a gift it was to recognize that blessing right then and there as it unfolded. I didn't have to wait for weeks for the serendipity of that "chance" meeting to hit me over the head. Right away I sat up and paid attention, immediately grasping what it was I was being taught.

In the 11 days I spent with Steve, I surprised myself and lost 6 pounds, but the weight loss was almost incidental to the lessons learned. My attitude, my outlook, and my commitment to my program was solidly restored. I came home feeling refreshed, and confident that I could continue with the step-by-step work I'd begun a year previous.

My mini-retreat was well worth the time and effort it took to coordinate cat-sitters, arrange for the lawn to be mowed, the mail to be picked up, the indoor plants to be watered, and have various other day-to-day tasks taken care of by my incredibly supportive local friends.

My do-it-yourself retreat was the best possible way I could have spent a portion of my summer vacation. And speaking of spending, I managed to save about $41,250 in the process, which made me an extremely happy woman.

Maggie and Miki revisited

Meanwhile, Maggie and Miki continued along their own paths to wellness. By July, the three of us had collectively lost just over 250 pounds, with approximately the same amount left to lose for all of us to attain our self-determined goals. To keep our motivation high, we started thinking about planning a "midway celebration."

"The last 250 pounds will be the hardest," I reminded them, tongue-in-cheek.

The second Sunday of October, Columbia Memorial Hospital sponsors an annual "Bridge Walk," spanning 10K, or a little over six miles, from the Washington to the Oregon side of the Columbia River, across the Megler-Astoria Bridge. We agreed to get together that fall to do the "Great Columbia River Bridge Crossing" as a three-person walking team.

But as soon as I began "training" in earnest, a nasty little bone spur on my left heel threw my well-intentioned plans into disarray. The heel spur was so painful that I couldn't walk more than a slow mile at a time, and some days not even that. I saw a succession of doctors, attended a series of physical therapy sessions, alternated heat and ice after exercise, with little improvement.

Undaunted, I registered for the Bridge Walk anyway. I figured my foot problems would surely be resolved in the more than two months before the walk, and three of us would joyously conquer the "challenging incline near the end," as the brochure referred to it, together.

Heigh-ho Silver, away!

"Auntie! Auntie!" My 10-year-old niece bounded across the front yard of her family's beach cabin and met me at my car door. "We're going to go ride horses on the beach! Wanna go with us?"

I looked into the bright blue eyes of my darling niece as I gave her a great big bear hug. How could I refuse anything she asked of me? "Sure," I said, "I'd love to."

But while "ride a horse on the beach" really *was* on my birthday resolution list of things to do that summer, I must admit it wasn't on my list for *that particular day.*

Five of us approached the registration table, money in hand, and the woman in charge surveyed our group, top to bottom and back again. Her eyes came to a stop on me. "Our horses don't carry more than 220 pounds," she said pointedly.

I felt a fast flush take over my whole neck and face. "Then I guess that lets me out," I said honestly, knowing I'd tipped the scale that morning at 265. I looked over at my sister—my niece's mother. She is a few inches taller than me, and carries her size well. I had no idea what she weighed at the time. "That lets me out too," she admitted. "I think we should all go check out one of the other horse rental places."

At our second stop we asked before they could embarrass us if there was a size restriction. The woman there quickly looked us over and said, "We have some larger horses for larger people. I don't see a problem here."

I let go the breath I'd been holding and we began filling out the liability release forms. "Horseback riding is classified as a Rugged Adventure Recreational Sport Activity," the form stated. "According to NEISS (*National*

Electronic Injury Surveillance Systems), horse activities rank 64th among injuries resulting in a stay at U.S. Hospitals. Related injuries can be severe, and may have lasting residual effects."

Did I really want to do this? I glanced at my darling niece. She was happily initialing all 12 of the individual release clauses, including the waiver for wearing a helmet. I certainly didn't want to disappointment her, yet I also didn't want to put myself in a position to foolhardily endanger myself because of my size.

"How long have you been renting horses on the beach?" I casually asked the woman in charge.

"Seven years," she told me, "and there's never been an injury," she added, anticipating my next question.

I completed the form and joined the group being paired up with their mounts. Quite obviously, they gave me one of the significantly larger horses. Fair enough. But this horse was *so large* I felt compelled to ask where they kept the beer truck it usually pulled.

"Those are Clydesdales," laughed the handler. "This is a Belgian quarter horse cross."

Small consolation. The horse had hooves the size of dinner plates, and a back so broad my legs stuck straight out on each side of him.

"His name's Trigger," she said.

"Trigger? As in Roy Rogers' 'Trigger'?"

The woman smiled. "He'll be gentle with you."

Gentle was not the word for Trigger. Comatose, maybe. He walked so slowly we soon fell quite a ways behind. I felt like a poor little fat girl who can't begin to keep up with her friends. One of the handlers rode back and suggested I "give him a little kick" so we'd catch up.

"Actually, we're doing just fine," I told her. "When the

group turns around, we'll have a head start."

She smiled, urged her own horse ahead, and suddenly Trigger decided he didn't want to be left back after all. He broke into a trot, and with this new advanced gait, I discovered I now had a tailbone. A tailbone that slapped painfully hard against the saddle with every jounce.

Reacting instinctively, I clasped my arms tightly across my chest to keep my big bouncing boobs from blackening both my eyes.

Whereas I had previously worried about my legs being ripped from their hip sockets, I shifted my concern to keeping upright.

"Auntie!" called my niece as I rejoined the group and Trigger resumed his one-speed-suits-all pace. "Are you having fun, like me?" She beamed.

"Probably not," I admitted between clenched teeth, "but I sure like being with you while *you* have fun!"

That was good enough for her, and she skillfully maneuvered her horse through the pack and back into the lead. I had to smile. She's quite a kid.

But my adventure was far from over.

Returning to the starting point, each rider was helped to dismount. Astride Trigger, who was just over 16 hands high, the ground appeared a very long ways away. I wasn't sure I could bend my knee far enough to get down without falling. "Could I have something to step off onto?" I asked.

They provided me with a green plastic beach chair. I hoisted my right leg over Trigger's rump, and stepped tentatively onto the seat of the chair. My left foot was still in the stirrup when Trigger decided to take a few steps forward. The chair tipped drastically, and my life flashed before my eyes. The last scene played out only in my overactive imagination—of me being dragged underneath the flying hooves of my marauding mount.

The reality was bad enough—the flimsy chair buckled and broke into a plethora of pieces. The words "mortified," "humiliated," and "devastatingly embarrassed" suddenly rushed into my panic-stricken mind.

And just as suddenly, my left foot popped free of the stirrup, and I miraculously stood upright in the soft sand.

I wanted to kiss the ground, but my darling niece pulled me by the hand toward her father, who'd wisely spent his hour listening to the radio in their truck. "Auntie!" she said, "Wanna go with us on the mopeds next?"

I wasn't about to tempt fate a second time that day. While a part of me desperately wanted to go with her, my rational mind knew my body was holding me hostage.

Maybe next year, I thought to myself as I opted to keep my brother-in-law company in the truck. Maybe next year.

A metaphorical fish tale

Sturgeon fishing on the Columbia River has always been a particular passion of mine. Other than being able to step safely on and off the boat, weight isn't particularly an issue in enjoying a day of fishing.

In the summer of 2000, I went out sturgeon fishing with friends on six different occasions. The peace, the serenity, the quiet of a day on the water quickly surrounded me with plenty of opportunity for genuine introspection and personal reflection.

On one excursion I considered how my weight loss program had a lot in common with reeling in a big fish. Once the hook is set, most fish will put up a hell of a fight, trying desperately to rid themselves of the force which is pulling them ever-closer to the waiting net.

Some fish, however, will try to fool you, swimming directly towards the boat, making you think they've already tossed the hook. Then, when there's enough slack in the line, they are often successful in spitting the hook out and making a clean get-away.

Following this train of thought, I mused one still hot summer afternoon, that surrender is actually the answer to the problem. If you fight it, you're doomed to be someone's dinner. If you let go and let God, you stand a good chance of the Universe stepping in and providing the perfect opportunity for you to receive the blessings that are unequivocally in your best interest.

The more you resist, the tighter the grip your obsession takes. It's a simple matter of willfulness versus surrender. In surrendering, you ultimately find strength.

Going for a test drive

By late August there were only two things left on my birthday resolution list: Test drive a Corvette, and fall in love. Who knew I'd accomplish both goals the same day.

John had entered my life via the Internet. He was smart, funny, good-looking, and best of all, he seemed to genuinely *like* me. We wrote daily emails for a month before deciding to meet. By that time we were talking on the telephone several times a day.

A certifiable romantic, John often called my answering machine while I was at work to play songs with words like "I knew I loved you before I met you" into the recorder for me to listen to when I got home.

Starved for love as much as food, I was swept away.

John and I came face to face for the first time on the Long Beach Boardwalk. The initial eye contact was electric. Although I felt a bit self-conscious at 248 pounds, it didn't seem to faze him a bit. At last I was free to be my true self with a man who appeared to adore me.

The fact that he arrived driving an '85 Corvette had nothing to do with my attraction to him whatsoever. None. Nada. Hunh-uh. Not a bit. The Corvette was just the sprinkles on the frosting of the cupcake of my happiness.

But—and there's almost always a but—John was in transition. Although he had maintained a separate residence for over a year, his divorce was not yet final. Truth be told, the paperwork for his divorce hadn't even been filed yet. He had quit his job of 15 years because his not-quite-yet-ex also worked there and he needed to distance himself. He was just a week or two into a new job when we met.

To top it off, his beloved brother had been killed in a car accident just days before he came to the beach for the first time. We'd been talking on the phone when he'd gotten the devastating call from his sister-in-law. He delivered his brother's eulogy earlier the same day he turned his car in my direction.

John was in transition all right, but so was I. My metamorphosis was occurring on a daily basis, and I was not sure who I was at any particular time. In our first few days together, I evolved from a rather insecure morbidly obese woman to a viable, dare I say sexy, heavier middle-aged woman. From thinking of myself as obese to merely being overweight was an incredible jump, and it left me with my head spinning.

But John had never known me any other way, and he accepted from the very beginning what I shared about my food plan and the work I was doing to further my program of recovery.

Yes, we ate out every meal, but we ate moderately and sanely and then spent the rest of the evening out dancing off the calories. Although my heel pain was anything but under control, I would have willingly walked on shards of glass for the opportunity to dance with him.

In a little over a year, I had gone from 396 to 248, a loss of almost 150 pounds, and to be able to wear a long dress and do a modified swing dance and the two-step and the waltz again was more than a dream come true. John was an excellent dancer, and I enjoyed every minute I was in his arms swaying to the music.

The first time we went out dancing, John had two drinks, then he handed me his car keys in front of several of my friends. All eyebrows went up. He didn't have another alcoholic beverage all evening, and he was certainly capable of driving us home himself, but he wanted me to know he trusted me without reservation.

Naturally, I was totally awed, not having been treated with so much dignity and respect in a very long time. I quickly fell head over heels for this charming and chivalrous man, and the drive home, behind the wheel of a Corvette, sitting next to the man I believed to be my Prince Charming, was, up until that time, the most exhilarating ride I had ever taken.

CHAPTER V:
ONE HUNDRED FIFTY POUNDS DOWN

Fatteningly ever after

John, John, John. My world, in the fall of 2000, revolved around John. A new school year started, but I hardly even noticed. My feet were barely touching the ground. I was ecstatic! Could this be love?

I began to obsess. When would I see him again? What was he doing when he wasn't with me? How long before he'd meet some skinny young thing? Where was he when he didn't answer his phone? How long until he invited me to come visit *him* for a change?

Yet our weekends together were magic. Magic, and much too short. We spent our time in a fantasy world. No day-to-day activities ever interceded. He made it clear from the beginning he wasn't here to tackle a "Honey Do" list during the weekends. His visits to the beach were strictly for his/our playtime!

So we went dancing, and then we came home and snuggled under the covers, but never any sex. I really wanted to have sex, and I even tried to initiate it several times, but he always held back, saying, "I'm too tired," or "Maybe in the morning," or "Let's not rush things," and I began to feel the familiar and painful pangs of insecurity telling me I wasn't attractive enough.

Whenever he visited, which was now about every other weekend, John insisted we go out to dinner. Never once did I actually cook a meal. That was okay with me; cooking was not high on my list of priorities.

John, however, had done the domestic thing with other women, and he enjoyed having the time and money to dine in nicer restaurants. Unfortunately, dining out still triggered my feelings that said I *deserved* to eat well, and often I ate more than I knew I needed if I wanted to maintain adherence to my food plan.

John went through the motions of supporting my weight loss efforts. At least he talked the talk. He even challenged me to a diet contest of sorts, suggesting that he could lose more than I did before we met again.

He lost that bet, by many pounds, as his weight went steadily up while mine continued slowly going down. It did not set well with him. He tipped the scale at about 250, and it was the first time in decades I'd dated a man who weighed more than I did. And although he said he was "trying" to lose weight, he wasn't following any kind of a food plan and he did not eat particularly health-promoting food. His frustration fueled his denial of his own eating and/or drinking disorder.

I wanted to be with him as often as possible, but unfortunately, when we were together, that meant I put my food plan on "hold." I became stalled at the crossroads. I realized we weren't long for this world if I didn't feel he was behind me and my weight-loss goals 100%.

Then quite suddenly, I saw signs of my former dealings with spousal sabotage lurking not far beneath the surface of our relationship. One night, as we finished a large, extravagant dinner, John ordered dessert. With two spoons. "Lighten up," he said. "Enjoy yourself. A couple bites won't kill you."

Where others had just begun

Somehow I managed to hover between 240 and 245 throughout September. I was in total denial about my relationship with John. I refused to see the forest for the trees. I obsessed constantly, alternately worrying if I didn't lose weight fast enough he would soon reject me, and then fretting if he didn't join me in my efforts to limit what I ate, I'd never be able to continue to lose any more weight at all.

Meanwhile, it didn't escape my notice that 240-something seemed to be the average starting weight for the now-slender women gracing each and every cover of Woman's World, a weekly magazine found at grocery checkout aisles.

Amateurs! I thought with some disgust. I'd already lost 150 pounds. What did any of these women know about being truly obese?!

Somewhere lurking in the far recesses of my brain I realized, with no small degree of pain in the acknowledgment, I now weighed where a "normal" fat person most often took back control.

Control. What an illusion! I was never, and would never be, in control. Food had always been in control. I knew I had to let go of these crazy thoughts if I ever wanted to be free from the constant obsession.

Fighting with myself was pointless. Wrestling the demon of compulsive overeating for 46 years had worn me out. I knew I had to surrender my will and my life to my

Higher Power. I absolutely, positively, had to let it go. Turn it over, and let it go!

As far as reaching my goal weight, I was still 80 pounds or so from what I would deem success. I became more resentful than ever of those I thought, in my narrow-minded and judgmental outlook, had no clue what it felt like to be mocked and ridiculed at every turn.

Depression settled over me. Although I called a few of my friends in the support group, I couldn't shake the overriding sense of hopelessness. I thought I was doomed to give in to my disease. I couldn't seem to grasp the handle on my current frame of mind.

Finally, I managed, one more time, to pick up that 2000-pound life preserver, also known as a telephone, and place a call to my beloved New York David. In his own indubitable way, he immediately set me back on the right track. He reminded me once again to look at how far I'd come, and to celebrate how many pounds I'd already lost.

"But David," I joked, "first I lost the equivalent of the petite little school secretary who weighs 115, bless her heart, then I lost your weight, at a measly 130 pounds, and now I'm working on losing Idaho Steve at 175." I sighed. "Pretty soon I'll be all alone."

"Relax," he reassured me, "I'm not going anywhere."

I took comfort in that thought. New York David had never met me face to face, but he had always been there for me and believed in me. To him at least, I was the same person I had always been.

"I want to ask you a question," he said, as we were winding up our conversation. "I want to ask you how it feels not to have me sitting on your lap all day. Do you feel better now without my entire weight hanging like a stone around your neck? Can you imagine carrying my entire body weight around with you every day?"

I pictured myself on the cover of Woman's World. Then I pictured David, all 130 pounds of him, sitting on my lap. I smiled. It was sure something to think about.

Fashion sense

"I know I need to break down and get some smaller clothes," I lamented to Maggie and Miki, my cohorts in weight loss, "but I don't want to spend a lot of money on things I consider 'temporary' and 'transitional'."

Miki, living 350 miles closer than Maggie, arrived at my door the next day with a large plastic bag stuffed full of clothes she could no longer wear. "You're now about the size where I started," she said. "Maybe some of these clothes will work for you. If you don't want them, please just drop them off at the thrift shop for me."

Some of them fit fine, some of them didn't, but bless her heart, she understood my dilemma and her compassion was gratefully acknowledged.

It's not that I was too cheap to treat myself to new clothes, I told myself, I was just afraid of not getting my money's worth before I lost enough to fit into the next lower size. Call me frugal.

Besides my frugality, I was faced with not knowing if I could, or should, buy clothes which had previously been "outside my comfort zone." For instance, at what precise weight is it considered socially acceptable for a woman to wear horizontal stripes in public?

And what about bright colors? "You don't paint a barn red," had been tattooed into my brain by well-meaning family and friends who also repeatedly informed me that "dark colors are slimming." Like you can trick someone into thinking a 396-pound woman is wearing a perfectly normal size if she's dressed like Johnny Cash? Get real.

Remember my wardrobe consisted of elastic-waist polyester stretch pants and a plethora of polyester pullover flower-print tops with three-quarter length sleeves. I was a true Polyester Princess.

In contrast, Miki described herself as a bit of a fabric snob. The clothes she brought me to try were either 100% cotton or soft slinky silk. There was even a light blue two-piece outfit in raw silk. Most of them were one solid color. There was nothing in my closet at the time that was one solid color except my slacks.

Heretofore, if it wasn't 'wash and wear' I didn't own it. 'Iron' was a foreign four-lettered word. And heaven forbid if there were buttons down the front. Buttons had a nasty habit of either coming *un*buttoned or gapping significantly across my chest, and I would go to any length to avoid *that* particular embarrassment, especially in front of a roomful of pubescent 7th grade students!

Yet a whole new world suddenly blossomed before my eyes. Unimagined colors, fabrics, and styles became accessible. Whereas I had worn only 'swishy-loose' tent-like blouses, I now began to wear some that disclosed the barest hint of a figure lurking beneath the material. I felt awe and pride when I bought a variegated lavender blouse with shoulder pads that had form-fitting darts running from the chest to below the waist.

I took a good hard look in the mirror. The woman in the mirror took a good hard look back. I didn't recognize her. Somewhere along the way I had morphed from being 'morbidly obese' to simply being 'fat.' Whether the politically correct euphemism was 'overweight', 'heavy', 'large', or 'plump', fat was fat, and right then I was quite happy to be so.

Realizing just how far I had come was certainly something to celebrate, so I celebrated by ordering many hundreds of dollars worth of new clothes from my trusty mail-order catalogs, including several long dresses.

Aborted Bridge Walk

"You can do anything you really *have* to do," Grandmother used to say.

"That's the problem," I said to myself, "I don't really *have* to do this." I sighed. "But boy-howdy, I sure *want* to." Desperately and passionately, the idea had consumed my waking moments for months.

"The Great Columbia Crossing," better known locally as "The Bridge Walk," happens only once a year, on the second Sunday of October. The year before I had pledged to be among those who completed the 10K trek. Ten kilometers translates into a little more than six miles, and this particular 10K boasts a "challenging incline," according to the promotional website, in the fifth mile. For us locals, that incline translated to one very long, very steep hill, lovingly referred to as "The Stairway to Heaven."

My friends Maggie and Miki and I planned this bridge-crossing odyssey together. Maggie lived in Walla Walla, but made special arrangements to have some time off, and Miki resided here at the beach.

The Achilles tendinitis I had developed in June continued to plague me. After x-rays confirmed the presence of a nasty heel spur irritating the tendon, the doctor set me up with a regimen of physical therapy. I began wearing cushions and lifts in all my shoes and practiced special stretching exercises morning, noon, and night. My compulsive zeal prompted friends to ask if I was training for the Olympics.

By mid-September I had been able to power-walk 2 ½ miles a day and optimistically sent in my $20 registration.

"I think I can. I think I can. I think I can," I chanted as I pushed the envelope. But envelopes, much to my dismay, can only be pushed so far. Applying ice after each workout soon failed to relieve the pain, which ran like electric shocks from my heel through my calf and deep into the tissue of my thigh.

"Why is this Bridge Walk so important to you?" asked my physical therapist, examining my swollen ankle two weeks before the big day.

It was a fair question. But how could I explain what my life had been like the previous year when I became breathless walking up a simple flight of six stairs? How could I express the drive and determination that hounded me week after week as I kept my eye on this goal? What words would convey the burning desire I had to bring my dream to fruition?

Eighteen months before this, Maggie and Miki and I had weighed a collective 372 pounds more than we did that autumn. That is not a typo. Using three different methods, or programs, the three of us had managed to release 372 pounds in 18 months. It was nothing short of a miracle. A true triumph of the human spirit.

To celebrate, I visualized the three of us climbing to the top of the bridge arch and symbolically hefting 26 fourteen-pound turkeys and a few odd giblets right up over the railing, cheering wildly as they plummeted down into the Columbia River. As I worked out all summer, this graphic image kept me smiling.

But I wasn't smiling the morning of the Bridge Walk. I also wasn't walking.

My heart ached as I watched Maggie and Miki board the bus to take them to the starting line. *This is so not fair!* I wanted to scream. *I trained hard for this day. I deserve to walk the bridge! I've earned this! Why isn't God paying attention? Life just sucks!*

But aloud, I simply wished them well and headed for the waiting area, tears stinging my eyes.

I took a couple deep breaths and slowly recited the Serenity Prayer: *God, grant me the serenity to accept the things I cannot change, the courage to change the things I can, and the wisdom to know the difference.*

Acceptance. Courage. Wisdom. Life's mammoth lessons all summed up in one tidy little prayer.

While I waited for my friends to enjoy "the thrill of victory," I had plenty of time to contemplate "the agony of de-feet." Yes, there were a few physical challenges for me still to overcome, but generally my health was so much better than a year before I consoled myself by looking forward to October 2001. God willing, Maggie and Miki and I would have a few more of those metaphorical turkeys to toss from the highest point of the Megler-Astoria Bridge.

I was proud of what my friends and I had thus far accomplished in our quest to reclaim our health and active lives. In my heart I knew all three of us had already beaten the odds to become undeniable winners. Intellectually, I absolutely believed this. Emotionally, I couldn't quite shake the feeling I'd failed.

Acceptance. Courage. Wisdom. Okay, I wasn't quite there yet; I'll always be a work in progress.

"Fiddle-dee," I said to myself as I watched the first few

people cross the finish line, "there's always next year." And I knew then the Great Columbia Crossing 2001 was not something I really *had* to do either, but boy-howdy, it was a goal I'd sure be aiming for.

Happy first anniversary

"I just called so you could sing 'Happy Birthday' to me on my dime," I told David on the tenth of October.

"Your birthday is in June," he replied matter-of-factly.

"Yeah, well, this is the day a year ago I was reborn," I explained. "It's the day I met you, and it's the day I began consciously abstaining from compulsive overeating."

"Then you mean it's our one year anniversary."

"Yes—I guess that's technically more accurate."

"Happy Anniversary, honey."

I smiled as I cradled the phone. "Happy Anniversary, David, my New York Angel, my Eskimo, my cheerleader. I couldn't have done it without you."

For a full year, David, the voice with the New York Puerto Rican accent, had been holding my hand as I rode the roller coaster through the trials and tribulations on my weight-loss journey.

For a full year he never once told me I was being foolish, or silly, or just plain dumb about my insecurities and concerns. He had listened, and accepted, and encouraged without faltering. He never told me he was "too busy" to talk, never put me down, never abandoned me.

There were no words to express how grateful I was.

"I love you, David."

"I love you too, honey," he replied without hesitation.

"And they say long distance relationships don't work." I

laughed. "I suppose if we ever met, we'd mess this up completely."

"We'll meet," replied David. "We have a date to go dancing. You're going to wear a red dress, remember?"

"I remember." I smiled again. "As soon as I get to goal, and my heel feels better, and I can scrape together the money to fly to the Big Apple, you can bet your booty we're going dancing!"

"I'm counting on it, honey."

"Me too, David, me too."

Dear John

Meanwhile, back in the real world of actual face-to-face relationships, all was not well. To all external eyes my liaison with John appeared to be steadfastly maintaining the status quo, but my gut told me there was plenty of big trouble lurking just beneath the surface.

Gradually, I came to realize I was compromising my own sense of self-worth, esteem, and potentially my food plan, by pretending nothing was amiss.

Too many sleepless nights and stomach-churning angst pushed me to compose a "Dear John letter" to dear John.

Dear John had never allowed me to visit him in his hometown, some four driving hours away, and although I investigated, and found out dear John had no other "main squeeze" living in that area, it was clear he did not want me as a part of his real life there.

"I've decided it would be best for my continued recovery to resign from the coveted position of "Queen of Unrequited Relationships," I wrote. *"No matter how we 'joke' about how you can't break up with someone you're not going with, or*

how we could each write a book on Commitmentphobia, or that a 90/10 relationship is no relationship at all, the bottom line is that we really aren't kidding, are we?"

It was the most difficult letter I had ever written, but I felt it was the only way to keep my weight loss equilibrium. I'd been eating to numb the pain again—the pain of believing in a relationship that didn't actually exist. I had given John incredible power over me, basing my happiness only on the condition of his validation, and now I wanted, and needed, my sense of balance restored.

While out walking on the boardwalk one morning at sunrise, I'd really listened to what my Higher Power was trying to tell me. I knew I didn't want to live my life as a hopeless codependent, and I was tired of feeling my life was "on hold," while I waited for someone else to tell me I was "good enough."

Instead, I made some tough choices. I chose to begin nurturing myself by committing only to a 50/50, or even better, a 100/100 partnership. I chose to honor myself by not falling in love with someone's potential. I chose to hold out for a person who values himself and his own health and supports those same ideals in me. I chose to remain food abstinent, and I chose to actively work the exercise program I had established for myself.

And in doing so, I also chose to let John go.

I thanked him for a wonderful August, September and October. I thanked him for showing me I could be a worthwhile, lovable, sexy woman, regardless of size. And I thanked him for all those emails, the spontaneous little phone calls, the dinners, the dancing, the flowers, but especially for the time we spent together. They were all truly wonderful memories.

I finished with some heartfelt words about timing being

everything, and the lessons we had both learned would certainly be a valuable asset to our continued growth, and then I wished him well and quietly said good-bye. No accusations, no blame, no guilt, no harm, no foul.

He did not respond, and that was just as well. I still suffered considerable backlashing fallout, however. It arrived in the form of the grand slam of all episodes of "consolation bingeing."

Consolation prize

If I couldn't have John in my life, at least I could have food. Food had always been there for me. When I had to cope with unpleasant feelings or uncomfortable situations, I had always known just where to turn.

The refrigerator didn't ask any questions. It didn't care if I opened the door with my eyes red and swollen from crying my heart out all night. Nary an eyebrow was raised if I hadn't bothered to get dressed all weekend.

My emotions were beyond raw. What was left of my spirit felt like so much pulverized hamburger. I was merely going through the motions of living. I ate to numb the incredible pain— to keep myself from feeling the true depth of my feelings.

I needed to be comforted in the worst possible way. But deep in my soul I also knew there wasn't a single problem in the whole world overeating couldn't make worse.

Once again, assisted by a power greater than myself, I picked up the 2000-pound life preserver. I called my best buddy in the support group.

"Help me," I barely choked out, "I'm relapsing."

"Not yet, you're not," she said. "By definition, a relapse

is a binge of many days or weeks or months—even years. A slip is just a day or two of compulsive overeating. By calling me, you have chosen to curb this behavior before it *becomes* a relapse. Good going!"

Good going?! Here I was, calling to confess I'd been shoveling food into my face fast and furious, for all the wrong (*were there any "right"?*) reasons, and she had the nerve to congratulate me?!

"This disease wants you dead," she continued. "Are you going to let it kill you, or are you going to surrender your willfulness and begin your abstinence again right now?"

If it kills me, I suddenly thought, *John wins.* And at the very same moment, I realized this had nothing whatsoever to do with John, and everything to do with my acceptance of things over which I had no control.

"I'll begin again," I told my friend, "right now."

"You go, girl."

But it wasn't quite that simple. I had written John off in early November. It was now a few days before Thanksgiving and I was hanging by my fingernails to a tentative and currently quite shaky program.

I declined invitations to join others for the traditional feasting day, even those who were following their own food plans. I didn't want my friends to feel they had to be my "food police." I stayed home and consoled myself further with much more food than necessary. I stayed home so I could sneak eat without witnesses.

"Pity party! Table for one!"

All I wanted to do was crawl into bed and pull the covers over my head. How in the world was I going to face the rest of the holiday season?

Catering by Costco

I mourned the end of my relationship with John for over a month, never managing to follow my food plan for more than three or four consecutive days, compulsively overeating for one or two or three days in between. I wondered if I would *ever* be able to return to my "before John" eating habits. I wondered if I would *ever* feel sane about food again.

Christmas quickly approached, and that meant it was time for my annual party. The previous year, with only two months of recovery behind me, I had sailed through the soiree without a single itty-bitty binge blip on the radar screen. This year, all bets were off.

Nevertheless, I planned and prepped my 17th fat-laden food fest just as if I weren't teetering precariously on the brink of total relapse. A creature of habit, I cruised the aisles of Costco, stuffing my shopping cart to maximum capacity with an eclectic assortment of frozen "just throw them in the oven for 12 to 18 minutes" hors d'oeuvres, just as I had always done.

During my support group meeting that week, I admitted that I was setting myself up for failure, but didn't know what to do about it without giving up the whole party idea, and I just wasn't willing to forfeit my traditional gathering. I felt I *had* to have the party, and therefore *had* to face down the food.

I heard myself playing a dangerous game of verbal volleyball, arguing for and against the celebration in alternate breaths. "I *love* Christmas. Without hosting this party the whole season will be ruined. I'm not about to let *my* food issues come between me and spending quality time with my friends." That statement was immediately followed by, "There's just too much temptation, too many calories in the food. There'll be too many opportunities to sneak eat, too many leftovers. I don't want this one isolated event to sabotage my entire life."

After the meeting, one of the women in the group quietly handed me a folded-over note. Inside was a copy of a prayer she said she recited every day. She said she hoped I would memorize it, and it would help me find the serenity of God's grace, both in my food and in my life.

The prayer goes:

"God, I offer myself to thee, to build with me and to do with me as thou wilt. Relieve me of the bondage of self, that I may better do thy will. Take away my difficulties, that victory over them may bear witness to those I would help of thy power, thy love, thy way of life. May I do thy will always."

I took the hand-written prayer with me to the beach and recited it over and over as I walked along the boardwalk. By the time I finished my 20-minute walk, I felt surrounded by a tangible and quite physical sense of calm. As soon as I got home, I pasted the prayer on the corner of my private bathroom mirror and vowed to read it morning and night. I fully surrendered myself to the words, and to the meaning behind them.

The party went off as planned. Much to my delight, it turned out it really wasn't about the food at all. It was about enjoying the company of friends and surrounding oneself in the love and comfort of God's grace on a daily basis— one day at a time.

I've often heard it said "Together we can do what we can never do alone," and I instinctively knew the loving support of the woman who handed me that prayer was a true Christmas gift from God.

All I want for Christmas

Miki flipped through the party pictures as we sat enjoying a cup of tea and the twinkling lights on the Christmas tree.

"So what did you ask Santa to bring you?" she asked.

"Santa doesn't need to stop here this year," I replied. "I had my Christmas when I had the party. The holidays are all downhill from there."

"I know what you mean." Miki smiled. "But if you *were* to ask for something, what would it be?"

I thought for just a moment before responding with deep sincerity. "A clavicle."

"*A what?*"

"A clavicle. You know, a collarbone. The bone on each side of your body connecting your neck to your shoulders. I've wanted to see my clavicle again for over a decade. There's been too much fat on my frame for me to see any sign or shadow of it, and I'm looking forward to that day."

Miki laughed. "Then today's your lucky day," she said. She flipped back through the stack of photos, and with great flourish, dramatically drew one out and placed it on the table in front of me.

The Christmas gathering had accidentally landed on the anniversary of the Boston Tea Party. On the invitations, I had suggested we all dress in colonial garb to commemorate the occasion. For my costume, I had dressed as a poor serving wench, complete with a lace-trimmed ruffled skirt, elbow-length bell-sleeved low-cut blouse, and white bonnet made from a curtain valance.

I looked at myself in the photo. Then I rubbed my thumb across the surface of the picture to make sure that what I thought I saw was real. There was, indeed, tangible evidence of my re-emerging clavicle. Emotionally overwhelmed, I choked up.

"You're looking a lot like the cat who swallowed the canary," said Miki.

I shook my head. "Too many calories in canary."

We both laughed and I looked again with awe and joy and gratitude at the picture in my hand. "Right now, instead of a poor little serving wench, I feel like I'm looking at The Wench Who Stole Christmas!"

Jim who?

"Finally!" said Mom when I answered the telephone a few weeks after New Year's. "I've been trying to reach you for days."

"Why didn't you just leave a message on the answering machine?"

"I wanted our conversation to be on my dime."

"It's a little more than a dime these days, Mom."

"Dime a minute with the phone card you gave me," she said, "so we'll talk fast. You can start by telling me why I never catch you at home anymore."

"I've been busy."

"Doing what?"

I hesitated. I shared most everything with my mother, but this time I'd been holding out on her for nearly a month. I took a deep breath before replying. "I've been going to the gym."

"You've been going out with Jim? Jim who?"

"I've been going *to* the gym, Mom, not with. *To* the gym. Gym's not a *who*, gym's a *what*."

"Doesn't he play second base?"

Trust Mom to turn our allegedly brief conversation into a rambling rendition of an old Abbott and Costello baseball comedy routine.

"Exercise more" was my number one resolution for the new millennium. Not that I *hadn't* been exercising. I'd been going to the pool twice a week and walking a mile or better whenever the weather permitted for over a year and a half.

Tacking "more" onto "exercise" only took four additional keystrokes, yet it made me rethink my fitness regime. What else could I do to hurry myself into a shapelier shape?

The answer was as obvious as the sign along the highway: "End Stress, Feel Happy, Be Healthy!" But actually getting out of the car and going through the door of the fitness center proved almost insurmountable.

I talked myself out of it a dozen times. With my medical history and physical limitations, what if there were no exercises I could safely do? What if the equipment wouldn't accommodate a person my size? What if I was too uncoordinated to complete a thorough workout? What if I totally embarrassed myself? What if I wore the wrong exercise clothes?

My "what if" list of concerns grew longer with each passing day, and I avoided making a commitment to try the gym out for several months.

As it turned out, I needn't have worried. Mike and Sharon, the proprietors of the fitness center, didn't laugh. They didn't even wince at my extremely less-than-buff condition. They exchanged no meaningful looks with each other as they signed me up and walked me through a beginning, beginning, beginners' routine.

I'd been afraid flexing my heretofore underused muscles might prevent me from lifting my toothbrush the next morning, but the fear went unfounded. After only one day's recuperation, I went back for another crack at the Nautilus instruments of torture.

Again, Mike patiently walked me through the seat adjustments and the weight settings and the number of repetitions and the proper form for using each machine.

And two days after that, I returned for Round Three. Yet again, with Mike hovering at my side, I moved from station to station, beginning with my warm-up, then the larger muscle groups, the smaller muscle groups, and on to my cool down.

Inside my head it began to be a game. I started wondering if I'd get taller by doubling my leg extension reps. I referred to the Hip Abductor as a Hip-Hip Away. The Abominable Abdominal machine dared me to increase the weight on my fifth visit, so I added 10 pounds then and 10 more the next week.

Through the miracle of technology, I discovered six minutes on the glider translated into 25 calories burned. Twenty-five calories is the equivalent of one half an Oreo cookie, or four and a half fat-free pretzel twists.

Settling in at four 45-minute sessions per week, I began to look *forward* to going to the gym. It must have had something to do with all those endorphins and serotonin and the other "feel good" natural chemicals being released into my bloodstream each time I exerted myself.

"It's almost scary," I told Mom. "At the ripe old age of 46, I've rediscovered the joy of exercise."

"What's scary," responded Mom, "is picturing my eldest daughter in fluorescent spandex."

"I don't wear spandex. This isn't that kind of place. I haven't even seen a bona fide yuppie. This gym's very friendly and comfortable."

"Which reminds me," said Mom, her tongue firmly planted in her cheek, "you still haven't told me much about your comfortable friend Jim."

"He's AnyBody's," I retorted. "AnyBody's Gym. Shall I tell him you said 'Hello'?"

"You be sure to do that," Mom replied.

Dining out

"Are you following Jared to Subway?" asked a friend I encountered while standing in line at our local sub shop.

"Jared who?"

"You know, *Jared...*" She pointed to a man's picture on a cardboard stand-up next to the cash register. "The guy who lost 245 pounds on the Subway diet."

Up to that moment, I had never heard of Jared. I'd been eating Subway sandwiches ever since the place opened locally, but I had gone there simply because it was another healthy alternative to cooking my own meals.

I had a mental list of all the places I could eat out and not compromise my food plan. When I went to the Lightship, I had Cobb Salad. At Chen's Chinese Restaurant, my favorite meal was Broccoli Chicken, sans rice. At the Potlatch, I dined on the cod filets and baked potato. I ate chicken frijitas at El Compadre, although I admit it was difficult to learn to refrain from indulging in the tortilla chip hors d'oeuvres. When in Astoria, I ordered the BK Broiler at Burger King without the mayo.

"Fast food" didn't have to be fattening, and eating out was one of the pleasures I refused to give up. Eating at home gave me too many excuses to prepare more than I needed and then avoid any possible leftovers by piling the food on my plate insisting it was "just one helping."

"It's all about making sane food choices," I told my friend. "I can eat anywhere I choose, as long as I remember to put my health first by ordering something compatible with my food plan."

"Well, whatever you're doing, it's certainly working," she said. "Jared would be so proud of you."

"Thank you," I replied. "I am proud of me, and that's really all that matters."

My friend then stepped aside and told me to go ahead of her. "I want to order just like you do," she explained.

I'd never received a greater compliment.

February madness

On February 12, I was 212 pounds. I noted that my weight exactly matched the date: 2-12. On Valentine's Day, 2-14, I was 214. Ok, I reasoned, it was probably just water weight. Never mind that the classroom Valentine party had raised havoc with my self-imposed sugar-free existence.

But by George Washington's birthday, 2-22, I had ballooned up to 222. What the devil was going on?

It was time to recommit, to rededicate myself to my health and my sanity. I called David, and then my friends in the support group, and then, although there were still a few days left in this disastrous month, I used a big, black felt marker and crossed February completely off the calendar.

Not waiting till the first of March, I immediately threw myself into making my pain-in-the-butt obsessive-compulsive nature work *for* me. I began using every tool at my disposal: I went to meetings, called friends, read support literature, followed my original food plan to the letter, wrote down every bite and I walked and/or went to the gym every single day, no excuses.

In three weeks I restored my sense of balance. But just when I thought it was "safe" again to relax my vigilance, I got thrown a triple-whammy curveball that sent me reeling.

It began with facing the fact head-on it was ridiculous to put off my heel spur surgery any longer. It was time to accept the things I couldn't personally change, but surgery could.

Every excuse for a binge

My heel spur bone removal surgery was scheduled for the end of March. As soon as the orthopedic surgeon and I set the date for the operation, the rest of my life imploded.

A quick check of the calendar told me I needed to schedule a dentist appointment before then, but my dentist of 23 years had recently died. The new guy in town couldn't see me for months and I was afraid before I was able to get in, I would pass the deadline to maintain maximum benefits from my dental insurance.

My life-saving counselor sent out form letters saying she was closing her private practice. I was quite sure I was nowhere near ready for her to discontinue helping me with this leg of my journey, and took it quite personally.

My Physician's Assistant, the woman who had sent me to that same kick-butt counselor two years previous, gave notice that her medical group was withdrawing from the area and she had decided this was the perfect time for her to move to Colorado.

One of my best friends, one of the first people I met socially when I moved to the beach 23 years ago, told me she had breast cancer and would be undergoing chemotherapy. My first thought was, "I'll kill you if you die!" but I kept *that* particular thought to myself.

My sense of abandonment threatened to overtake what little sanity I clung to. I had to remind myself again and again the world did not revolve around *me, me,* and *only me.* I felt bitter and put-upon and resented all these things "happening to me" at the worst possible time. I wanted to eat, eat, and eat some more, but I recognized the food triggers and managed to remain abstinent day-by-day, hanging on by the tippy-tips of my chewed-on fingernails.

To add one more thing to my beyond-the-danger-level stress load, my principal made it clear she was none too pleased that I'd be missing 15 days of school for my heel surgery. Never mind I had conscientiously scheduled the operation for the day *after* I would have third quarter grades entered into the computer, or that my recovery time encompassed all of my precious spring break, or that I was committed to being back to work full time before the 7th graders had formal state testing or conference week—she was still not happy with my timing.

"Can't you wait until summer?" she asked.

When I assured her I could not, she then remarked, "If you didn't go out dancing every weekend, you wouldn't need this done at all."

I hadn't been able to dance in over six months, but she hadn't known that. I *wanted* to be able to dance again. I wanted to be able to *walk* without pain again, and the doctor and I both felt we had exhausted all other alternatives, including months of physical therapy, heel pads, arch lifts, special exercises, even herbal supplements. Surgery was my very last resort; I wanted the 80% chance of being "pain free" after the six to nine months the doctor told me I'd need to commit to full foot recovery.

The Sunday before surgery, I sat at my computer and began to type out my Last Will and Testament. Any time a person has major surgery, even a planned-for surgery, there's a risk involved, and I was not real crazy about being under general anesthetic for a couple hours. I'd had trouble waking up from anesthetic before, and things happen. So to me, writing my Will that Sunday afternoon was a kind of quasi-insurance policy—if I were "prepared" to die, then of course I'd live.

But a funny thing happened as I typed out my bequeaths. I began to see just how much "good" could result from my death. I acknowledged a lot of people could pay off bills, take vacations, finish school, put down payments on cars, and in other ways benefit from me leaving them a few thousand dollars each. Perhaps it was God's plan that I was "supposed" to die.

And if I was going to die anyway, then there were some things I wanted to eat first—

The closest "food" to the computer was within easy reach. I didn't even have to leave the room. I had stored numerous bags of Easter candy in my home office to make little treat baskets for all 128 of my 7th grade students. The candy had been there for weeks and hadn't bothered me a bit. Until now.

With tears in my eyes, already mourning my own demise, I ripped opened a jumbo-sized bag of colorful malted milk ball Easter "eggs." I poured some into my hand and popped them into my mouth. I hardly tasted them as I chomped a few times and swallowed.

I continued working on the finer points of my Will. Type two or three lines, eat five or six malt ball eggs. Type a little more, eat a few more. The afternoon and evening passed by as I alternately cried and binged.

By the time I finished writing, I had also finished one entire bulk bag of candy. It was then and only then that I read the "nutritional label" on the back of the bag.

There were 180 calories in a "serving" of malt ball eggs. A "serving," according to the label, consisted of 8 pieces of candy. There were "approximately" 33 servings in the bag.

I knew better, but I did the math anyway. Thirty-three times 180 calories tallied up to a whopping 5,940 calories. And this was in addition to all my "regular" food consumed that day! Six thousand calories equated to roughly *four days* of my regular food!

I ran to the bathroom, leaned over the toilet and stuck my finger down my throat. Nothing happened. I tried two fingers. Nothing. I tried using my toothbrush to gag myself. Still nothing. I put the lid down on the commode, sat down, and cried buckets of tears.

When I finished with my self-inflicted pity party, I stood up and washed my face. I looked in the mirror. Mathematically, I knew that 6,000 calories should not amount to even a two-pound gain. But emotionally, I freaked out at the potential devastation a sugar binge like this could do to my program.

Taped on the mirror was a poster instructing "How to Love Yourself" by Louise L. Hay, author of "You Can Heal Your Life." The poster had been given to me by my best support group buddy. Although I read the words often enough, I was moved again by their simple encouragement.

The next day I was 100% back on my program. When I went into surgery a few days later I weighed 210 on the hospital scale. I hadn't weighed 210 for almost 13 years. And 210 was just 11 pounds from having a *one* in the first digit. It was exactly the kind of motivation I needed for me to vow "not to gain" during the weeks or months I would be unable to walk or do much else in the way of exercising. A vow I kept, and then some.

Some pain, but no weight gain

My heel spur was removed the last Friday in March and I came home the same day. I was completely "non-weight bearing" for the first two weeks, then advanced to a fiberglass cast (*I chose a purple one!*) with a boot-like "shoe" to begin hobbling around on, slowly weaning myself from dependence on crutches.

Two weeks later, still in a great deal of constant pain, and still using crutches for balance, I returned to work. My return date had been carefully planned so I would be back a couple days before the 7th graders had a week of mandatory state testing, so as to minimize disruptions in their daily routine.

When I went back to work near the end of April, the first thing I did was step on the nurse's scale. I weighed 205, *with the cast on!* I had lost five pounds during my month of immobility. I was very pleased, and perhaps a little too cocky.

Thursday of that week was "Conference Day," in which teachers worked from 7:45 a.m. until 7:00 p.m. to accommodate working parents. There was a scheduled dinner break, and take-out food was delivered to the Home Economics room. Unfortunately, there were no choices. Dinner was an assortment of thick-crust pizza and chocolate frosted brownies for dessert.

I had not prepared myself for this encounter with known trigger foods. Had I known what the menu included ahead of time, I would have hidden in my classroom and eaten more appropriately. I hesitated a second too long, and the smell of hot fresh pizza quickly dissolved any possible resistance my hungry stomach might muster.

As it was, I succumbed in the worst possible way. My "Pizza pig-out and brownie binge," as I later referred to it, did not end at the conclusion of the dinner break. Shortly after 7 p.m., as soon as I could leave the building, I headed straight for the McDonald's drive-thru window.

I ordered a large Butterfinger "McFlurry" to satisfy my sudden and desperate craving for ice cream. Rationalizing that "I've blown today already," I compounded the problem by dumping in several hundred more calories. "It's part of the dairy food group," I told myself, as if that really mattered.

I finished wolfing down the frozen treat just in time to pull into my favorite "31 flavors" stop. Tightly clasping a double-scoop waffle cone in one hand, I drove on towards home, as out of control with my food obsession as I had ever been in my entire life, and that was saying something!

But I wasn't through, even yet. At the last market before leaving town, I propped what was left of my cone in the car cup holder and went in to buy several more ice cream bars. I considered M&Ms and Hershey bars as well, even stood at the check-out counter with them in my hand, but my craving right then was focused on ice cream rather than candy and I didn't have enough cash with me to buy both.

By the time I arrived home, the sugar rush had me flying higher than a kite. I felt totally nauseated. I wanted to purge, but again, I couldn't make myself throw up no matter how many fingers I stuck deep down in my throat.

Nearing 9 p.m. I don't know how I managed it, but somehow I picked up the phone and called my accountability partner from the weekly support group. She didn't condemn, didn't judge, and wasn't the least bit critical. "What's done is done," she said. "Now tell me what you plan to eat tomorrow."

I committed my food for the next day to her right then and there, and by the grace of God, I stuck to it.

CHAPTER VI:
200 POUNDS DOWN:
"Oh my God! The first digit is a one!"

Scaling down

Although I knew better, I weighed myself every day, morning and night, for several weeks, rationalizing I didn't want to miss "the big event." I wanted to know, and fully appreciate, the *exact moment* when the scale confirmed the existence of my Higher Power. (*As if by now there was any doubt of His work being done!*)

I had not been so obsessed with weighing before, but now stepping on the scale was the first and last thing I did each day. Okay, to be absolutely truthful, it wasn't the *very* first thing I did in the morning. Naturally, I had to use the facilities first. Because, as everyone whose ever tried to lose weight knows, every single ounce counts!

And speaking of "extra ounces," I was now wearing a hard black plastic removable cast on my left foot. I took it off for sleeping and bathing, *and weighing myself,* but it would be some time before I could walk without the extra support and stability it gave me.

I tottered to the bathroom each morning and gently stepped on the scale, hoping today would be the day, yet it seemed I was purposefully throwing little hand grenades at myself to keep from achieving my goal.

One day I ate *two* bags of fat-free microwave popcorn. And while it's true the popcorn was included on my "legal" food plan, it's also true it contained a high amount of salt. And sodium in any form makes some small amount of water retention a certainty. "It's not about the numbers" I kept telling myself, but I knew inside I really, *really* wanted to see those numbers keep moving down.

Following an abstinent food plan, regularly exercising, and simply the passage of time, will eventually bring forth the desired results. It's what I had bet my entire life on.

My payoff arrived on a beautiful spring Thursday. May 3, 2001, to be exact. Another day that will live in infamy.

As I expelled every bit of air from my lungs and oh-so-softly stepped onto the scale, I already knew. Way down in my toes, I knew, with absolute certainty, today was *the day*.

Lo and behold, the numbers on the dial confirmed it. There was just a smidgen of a space where I could see the white background between the needle and the big black line delineating the 200-pound mark. And the 200-pound mark was *to the right* of the needle!

I was *under* 200 pounds. For the first time since 1982, I was *under* 200 pounds! I stood very still and savored the moment. Tears rolled off my chin and splatted on the floor. I laughed as I caught myself wondering how many tears it would take to shed another pound!

Then it occurred to me: At 198 pounds, I had *lost* 198 pounds. *I was half the woman I used to be!* My laughter rocked the scale and I was afraid to recheck the numbers, knowing my mirth had wiggled the needle, and I was not about to tempt fate.

Without looking down again, I stepped off the scale and put it away in the cupboard. I'd seen the promised land, and knowing how my weight could fluctuate 4 or 5 pounds *a day*, decided that it was in my best interest to try not to weigh again for several weeks.

I turned on the shower. Glancing in the mirror, I acknowledged a rather self-satisfied and smug smile. Okay, it was a bona fide smirk. It occurred to me that of us four siblings, I was now the only one under 200 pounds. *"HALLELUJAH!"* I hollered at my reflection, whirling my arms around over my head and grinning like a Cheshire cat. *"HALLELUJAH,* Girlfriend, you're a bona fide miracle!"

In just under two years, I had gone from the biggest kid in the family, to the smallest, and I still had a ways to go to be considered "normal." I offered a silent prayer for those in my family who might someday also choose to surrender their compulsive eating, and I thanked God for the progress that had been made in my own life thus far.

As I stepped into the waiting shower it felt as if the water baptized and confirmed the transformation in my life. Truly grateful for the experience of having this second chance, I washed away a little more of the wreckage of my past and was born anew.

Shape-shifting

My orthopedic surgeon released me to return to the gym "whenever you feel you can," on one condition. Although the doctor and I had a rough timetable for weaning me away from the removable cast, my visits to the fitness center were not included in that schedule. Inside the gym, the cast stayed on.

The recumbent bike enabled me to rev up my heart rate and burn a lot of calories at the same time. It did not require me to stress the heel in any way. The bike became my alternative to the "before surgery" walks. I longed for the day I could trek up and down the boardwalk again, but until then, the bike gave me the cardio workout I knew I needed to continue getting fit.

My friends at the gym were extremely supportive. They helped me adjust seat settings and started me back at much lower weights than I had lifted six weeks before. But the "muscle memory" was still there! Those three months of attendance at the center before my bone spur surgery paid off in spades. In just a few weeks I was able to add 10 pounds to almost every piece of equipment I was using, and a few weeks later further increased most of the weights by another 10. I was ecstatic! Cast bound, but ecstatic!

The only disappointment was the fact that my body weight had hit a very solid plateau and not budged since my return to the gym.

"You're shape-shifting," said a friend of mine.

"Shape-shifting?" I laughed. "You mean like on Star Trek? You mean I'm morphing into some new kind of celestial being? Cool!" I grinned wickedly. "Do I get to choose my new color, too? You know I've always wanted to have purple hair!"

She rolled her eyes and sighed. "Get serious! You know muscle weighs more than fat, right?"

"Right."

"And you know you've been really busy building back your muscles. Now I'm not saying that your whole body had atrophied or anything, but I bet you're firming up and losing inches instead of pounds."

As soon as I got home, I got out the tape measure. Sure enough, my friend was right, and if I'd been paying more attention, I would have known this all along. The clues were all there, starting with how well my clothes fit.

For several weeks, I had been fastening my bras on the inside hooks. I had *thought* the elastic in them was wearing out and I was only taking up the slack from their apparent relaxation of support.

In reality, my bust measurement had gone down two inches since before my foot surgery. My waist and hips had also trimmed up a little, but I had plenty of underwear in various sizes so I never paid much attention to them.

Now I knew I had to break down and buy myself a couple new bras. I carefully retook the top, center and lower measurements and got out my trusty mail-order catalog to "do the math."

The great bra-buying ordeal

I carefully calculated my "new and improved" bra size using the chart in the center of the mail-order catalog and turned to the pages with the pictures of available styles. I found the brand I was wearing and circled the nine-digit number for easy reference when I placed the call.

But then I noticed something very odd. The bra sizes did not include the one I thought I needed. I was shocked to discover the sizes for my usual brand and style began with sizes *larger* than what I wanted!

In two years I had gone from wearing a 52FF to a 44DD and was using the innermost hooks to fasten it. Now I hoped that a 40DD would be sufficient to adequately support "the girls."

I scanned the pictures and descriptions of similar foundation garments. None of them had what I considered "my new size" bra; all of them began with 42s or larger.

I felt my emotions flash across my face like a kaleidoscope. My initial reaction was delight. Never had I *dreamed* I would be "too small" to order from my collection of trusty full-figure catalogs. On the other hand, I dreaded having to go to a store to try on bras of any size. I had shunned the whole dressing room experience for so many years, I didn't know quite what to expect.

The outlet mall in Seaside had a store completely dedicated to undergarments. I nearly turned around and left as soon as I walked through the door. So many choices! Colors! Styles! Brand names! How would I ever be able to narrow down the options to find a bra that would comfortably fit me?

I stood still and slowly scanned the whole room. I had been ordering "Goddess" through the catalogs, but there wasn't a section for that brand. I walked over to the Playtex 18-hour display like I knew what I was doing. (*Hey, if it was good enough for Jane Russell, I was pretty sure it was good enough for me.*)

Beige bras had been my standard, and I saw no reason to change now. That narrowed it down a little. I detested "underwire," so those were out. I knew I still needed wide straps, but it looked like that meant four hooks in the back instead of three. But maybe not.

I finally settled on a style, I picked out three different sizes. One I thought would be "too big," one I figured would be "too small," and a middle one that I figured would fit "just right."

The dressing room was adequately large, and had a full solid built-in bench to sit on along one wall. The opposing wall was one huge mirror. I'd never been a big fan of mirrors, but I reluctantly acknowledged the necessity of a "shows all" reflection here.

First I pulled on the bra I thought was "too big"—and it really was! I smiled a rather self-satisfied little smile and decided to try the "probably too small" one next.

This "probably too small" bra actually went around me just fine. In fact, as I looked into the mirror I realized that it would have fit if there hadn't been so much loose skin hanging over the tops and sides of the garment.

And there was loose skin everywhere. When I held my arms straight out from my body, the skin rolled over the side of the bra under my arm a full four inches, completely obscuring any view of the material. The cup of the bra sufficiently covered my actual breast tissue, but over the top hung a plenitude of extra "flab." I tried tucking it in, and it just oozed out elsewhere.

I freaked out. My breathing became shallow and I began to sob uncontrollably. I stared into the mirror and my reflection mocked me by jiggling and flopping all around. I sat down on the bench behind me, picked up my blouse, wadded it up, and held it over my mouth to increase my carbon dioxide in an effort to stop hyperventilating. I thought I might faint, and I bent over to put my head down closer to my knees, all the while crying my eyes out.

I had heretofore not confronted the concept that I might *never* get back the body I once had. In my naiveté, I thought once I took the numbers off the scale, I'd be the former high school athlete revisited. All this loose, hanging skin was not something I had imagined in any of my dreams about reclaiming my body and life.

The store clerk tapped softly on the dressing room door. "Are you okay in there?"

"No," I choked out, "but I'll be finished in a few minutes."

"Do you need me to get another size for you?"

"No, thank you," I replied, "I have more than I need."

"Are you sure you're okay?"

I wanted to point out to her I had never said I was "okay," but I let it pass. I reluctantly pulled on the "middle bra," the one I had originally thought would fit best, and reluctantly conceded it fit fine enough. The smaller-cupped bra had been a pipe dream to begin with, I told myself, but the unexpected pain of seeing that it fit, and yet didn't fit, was deep and penetrating.

I bought several of the "middle-sized" bras, all in the same boring color and style and brand, and left the store with swollen, puffy eyes. Outside, I took a deep breath and tried to shake the whole thing off.

Turning toward my car, I discovered two doors down I could get the medication I thought I needed to alleviate my pain: "The Rocky Mountain Chocolate Factory."

The sign shone like a Greek siren luring me closer to the rocks. In some kind of a weird drama-induced trance, I heeded their call. Once inside the candy shop, the familiar scent of deep, dark, bittersweet chocolate tantalized my nostrils. I could already taste it.

What happened next is still a little hard to believe. Somehow, someway, God took time out from His busy schedule, and walked into that chocolate shop with me. It must have been God; there's no other even semi-plausible explanation. And together God and I stood and smelled the wonderfully enticing smells of thick, rich brownies and cookies and hand-dipped decadent truffles. And then God whispered, "*You are not alone.*"

Well, I knew I wasn't alone, because there were several people in line at the counter ahead of me. My mouth watered, and I took another deep sniff of the palpable chocolate air. And God said, "*There's no problem in the world that eating sugar right now won't make worse.*"

I started to tremble. The people ahead of me gathered up several small bags of goodies and stepped aside.

"May I help you?" said the woman behind the counter.

I nodded, swallowed, and licked my lips. "Yes." Then my eyes focused on the display of stuffed animals behind her. "I'd like that Beanie Baby," I said, pointing to a newly-released Ty bear.

"Will that be it?"

"Yes," I replied, "that's all I need here today."

I paid for my purchase and was back in my car before I read the nametag of the Beanie Bear who had rescued me. It ruefully entered my mind that the bear's name should be "Goldilocks," as in "this bra is too big, this bra is too small, and this bra fits good enough."

As with all Ty Beanie Babies, the heart-shaped ear tag included the toy's name and a poem. The four-line poem read: "You give me hugs when I am sad; You love me if I'm good or bad; Thank you for all you do; I can always count on you!" The bear's name was "Hero."

Tears rolled down my cheeks one more time that day. "Thank you, God," I said aloud, and clutched my bear tightly to my chest. "*Thank you, God! Thank you, Thank you, Thank you!*"

Birthday burn-center blues

My dear friend Maggie and I were both born in 1954. However, since I was born a full three months before her, she often called in June to remind me of my rapidly advancing age, while she remained "a year younger" for the summer.

"So what do you want for your birthday?" she asked.

I sighed. My bra-buying ordeal was still a fresh and painful memory. "A lot less of this loose hanging skin," I replied despondently.

She echoed my sigh. "I just happen to have been looking into that very topic on the Internet a few days ago," she said. "Don't forget I have the same problem."

How could I possibly forget? During the two previous years, by entirely different methods, both of us had successfully trimmed our body size by more than half, and we were both nearing our self-determined goal weights.

"I was hoping to find a burn center that would pay a hefty percentage for the skin removal surgery," she continued. "The expense is incredible, and naturally, the surgery is most often deemed 'cosmetic.' Therefore, it isn't covered by insurance. I figured since burn centers always need more skin, and God knows I've got lots more skin than I need, maybe there's a program already in place to help with the cost."

"Count me in," I told her. "See if we can get a bigger discount if we have it done at the same time and share a hospital room."

"I'll email my research to you," she said. "But I'll warn you ahead of time, it's not very encouraging."

"Not very encouraging" was a gross understatement. The first article she forwarded contained information about general skin grafts. According to this report, many "skin banks" allegedly sold skin to the highest bidder, and cosmetic "enhancements," such as penis enlargement, often claimed the skin that might otherwise go to a burn victim.

Okay, I thought, now we know the skin must be designated to go to a specific burn center, not a skin bank. No problem.

The second article was unsettlingly graphic. It explained how skin was "harvested" from cadavers, one thin layer peeled away at a time. It was a very educational story, and I read it several times in its entirety, but I must admit I was greatly relieved that the article contained no pictures accompanying the text.

Next I read skin banks *preferred* to get skin directly from corpses rather than from tummy-tuck or other patients because there were no "additional expenses" of the hospital surgical suite, surgeon, or anesthesiologist.

Furthermore, skin retrieved from live patients had to have the epidermal layers "separated" from the fat and other tissue after harvesting, and it then had to undergo rigorous medical testing before it could be used. Apparently skin from dead donors wasn't subjected to such stringent tests or waiting periods before it could be reapplied.

All I'd been worried about up to this time was whether or not I had too many stretch marks for my skin to be viable, and now I was smacked in the nose by what I deemed "too much information."

"Let's not give up," said Maggie when next we chatted. "Maybe if we write a really good letter to Oprah, and tell her about all the weight we've lost, maybe she will help us pay for the surgery. Surely, *she*, of all people, would understand."

"Before you go writing any letters," I replied, "let me look a little deeper into this surgery stuff. I'm not too keen on the idea of going under general anesthetic for long periods of time; I have a history of trouble returning to the real world."

"Okay," said Mags, "I'll talk to my regular doctor about it at my next check up, and you can look into it from the cosmetic surgeon's standpoint."

"Deal," I said, and wrote "check out tummy tucks" on the top of my summer's "to do" list.

The dating game

Meanwhile, as a certified charter member of the non-existent west coast branch of The Lonely Hearts Club, I began to think it was about time to dip my toes back into the shallow end of the dating pool.

Six months and 50 pounds had elapsed since my sojourn with John, and summer was once again upon us. Thoughts of a sultry summer romance dominated my waking moments until I finally decided to take the plunge and write myself an attention-getting personal ad.

Heretofore I had only answered the online ads of others. It was probably yet another manifestation of my issues of "control." Previously, I had spent much time reviewing the ads with critical scrutiny before choosing to respond with a rather generic email 'hello.' If there was anything in a man's ad which even *remotely* suggested he was looking for a "slim, trim, petite, attractive, active, svelte, etc., etc.," Barbie-doll type, I didn't bother to reply.

Most guys' initial replies to my brief hello provided me with enough information to opt to continue writing, or quickly press Delete.

I set up a separate webmail account for such encounters, untraceable by most casual users of the Internet. I had a fake name, fake address, a whole fake persona to keep my tracks covered and be "safe," until I decided the guy I was writing to was fairly legitimate.

But this time I decided to put myself "out there." Well, not really "myself," yet close enough that any "decent" guy would understand my caution if and when it became time to come clean about my true identity.

"Coastal Creature seeks Intelligent Male Life Form," read the subject line. And then I wrote a little about myself, and the dearth of educated, articulate men living in such a small gene puddle. "Non-smoker, non-drinker, college-educated and employed," I wrote, "seeks same."

"Be careful," said my friend Lee, after perusing what I'd written. "You're likely to get a couple dozen idiots trying to prove they're not stupid."

"And maybe," I countered, "just maybe, Prince Charming has been waiting somewhere behind the sand dunes for me to make my whereabouts known. I think I'm about ready for a real relationship. I'm ready to take a couple calculated risks."

"Go for it," said Lee, "but watch your back."

And to some extent, Lee was right. The first week the ad was online, I received numerous replies, many of which contained numerous spelling and grammar errors, politically incorrect points of view, or sexually explicit and/or suggestive information. Not that I *minded* the suggestion of sex, but there is a time and place, and a first email is definitely neither the time nor the place!

However, there were a couple men worth checking out, and I responded to those. I even met two of them face-to-face. But no "Love Connection" transpired.

The second week I received three more inquiries, but no keepers. The one man I met that week accompanied me on a tour of the area, and in a local gift shop we were approached by a former student of mine who happened to work there. "*WOW!*" she exclaimed, coming up and giving me a hug, "where's the other half of you?"

My escort stopped in his tracks and gave me the old

"elevator eyes," slowly looking me up and down a couple times. "I take it you used to be heavier?" he asked.

In my ad, I had described myself as 5'6", brown hair, brown eyes, and "HWP," which is the personals ad code for "Height/Weight Proportionate." What difference did it make what I *used* to look like? But I knew by his expression, that even if I had *wanted* to see him again, which I didn't, it wouldn't have been an option.

The third week, when I'd about given it up as "a noble experiment," I got an amusing, intriguing, and rather lengthy letter. The man was obviously educated, well-versed in many subject areas, sympathetic to my political and religious persuasions, and identified completely with my frustration in finding a suitable mate swimming in my "small gene puddle."

We began an intense and informative email correspondence, followed by hours of telephone calls, and shortly thereafter decided to meet "live, and in-person."

After an hour or so, my gentleman friend looked at me and said, "Well, do you like what I see so far?"

I cracked up. "Do you realize what you just said?" I asked him, and repeated his Freudian slip.

He didn't blush, but he squirmed just enough to give me the upper hand, which for some reason I didn't press. Instead, I simply smiled. "Yes," I replied a heartbeat or two later, "I am very pleasantly surprised."

The next time I met my new friend, I had accumulated 412,632 reasons why "this relationship can't work." My new friend agreed. Not the least of which, he told me, was the fact I "didn't fit his image."

Now hold on! I thought. It was one thing for *me* to come up with excuses for cutting and running, but what exactly did he mean by *his* remark?

"You're a wonderful woman," he began, "and you'd be absolutely perfect if you weren't so large."

If I weren't so large??!! What the hell did he know about what constituted LARGE?

"I'm looking for a woman around 130 pounds," he continued.

I used to have a leg that weighed that much! I thought.

Somehow, I kept my indignant ire to myself. I took a deep breath. And then another. When my respiration returned to a somewhat normal rate, I said softly, "And do you truly believe the quality of a woman's character can be determined by the size of her clothing?"

He didn't meet my eyes, and he didn't answer my question. Instead he replied, "I like spending time with you. I enjoy your companionship. As I see it, either you will change to fit my image, or my image will change to fit you, or we will eventually part company. But I'd like to continue getting to know you and see what happens."

I took another deep breath. *At least he's honest*, I thought. *And honesty counted for something, didn't it?* "Well, I'm looking for three things," I told him. "Passion, humor, and unconditional acceptance."

"I can give you humor," he replied with a straight face.

Of course, I busted out laughing.

"And you *deserve* all three," he went on, without a trace of a smile. "But only time will tell."

Only time, I thought, and right then I decided I didn't need to push this particular moment to a pivotal crisis point. I made a conscious decision to give it some time, just enough time, to see just what lessons God had in store for me. *Fasten your seatbelt*, I thought, *you could be letting yourself in for a pretty bumpy ride..."*

Sound the retreat!

It was June, and time for me to "go away for awhile." The year before, I had created my own "mini-retreat" at my friend Steve's in Idaho. Again, I turned my eyes eastward and planned my hiatus with a focus on continued commitment to my program and my evolving life.

Months before, at the suggestion of my kick-butt counselor, I had obtained workshop materials from the International Clarity Institute, Inc., in Madera, California. I hadn't yet opened the mammoth notebooks, rationalizing that I needed a dedicated period of uninterrupted time to tackle such a daunting project.

Now I packed the materials from the Institute in my "Retreat Box" and made this path of emotional healing the top priority for my trip.

Much of my Emotional Clarity work during my three weeks in relative solitude is too painful and too personal to recount. I faced my issues of having been told I'd "never be good enough" by people closest to me, and wrote volumes filled with anger and resentment toward people I have no intention of ever crossing paths with again. I needed to "let it go" and get on with my life, but first I had to acknowledge exactly what it was I was "letting go."

Day after day the venom surfaced. When I began this "emotional clearing," I had no idea I harbored such varied and bitter feelings. It was difficult for me to isolate and stick with each issue as it came up. I had to remind myself time and again that I was doing this work "voluntarily" and that intellectually, I knew, beyond a shadow of a doubt, that I would emerge a better, and more balanced, human being.

If I emerged.

Each morning, as soon as Steve went to work, I went

into rebellion mode. I imagined myself kicking and screaming while being dragged to the gallows. It was just a workbook, I told myself. I didn't have to face down all these demons at this particular time of my life. "Ignore it, and it will go away" became my battle cry and credo.

I wanted to run far and fast, both emotionally and physically. I found excuse after excuse not to sit down at the table and open the book each morning. I surfed the channels on the television. I rented mindless videos. I attended all sorts of "support group meetings," whether I wrestled with that particular addiction or not, just to keep my mind off my primary retreat goal.

I prayed constantly for the willingness to face whatever was left to be faced. And eventually, ever-so-slowly, I forced myself to sit down to answer just a few of the questions posed with honesty and openness.

Much of what I discovered made me extremely uncomfortable, but by the grace of God, I kept going. Little by little, I peeled away the onion layers of self-deception to the naked and quite vulnerable person left standing there.

Thankfully, I discovered I wasn't such a "bad" person after all, I just needed to be kinder and gentler with myself and begin nurturing the child who'd been hiding behind the hundreds of excess pounds for so many years.

There were many tears and much stomach upset throughout this self-discovery process, and I am grateful I had the time and opportunity to dig down and explore my emotional roots. As a direct bi-product of this work, I started taking tangible proactive actions. Change was in the air! Metamorphosis was upon us! Time for the butterfly to emerge from the cocoon!

I took my removable cast off and left it off. I began carefully walking short distances without it. I bought myself some new, much smaller-sized clothes, including several pairs of *jeans* for the first time in decades. Jeans that zipped up in the front and had no elastic! Then I called my hairdresser, long distance, and told her it was about time to get that gray out of my hair. Next I made an appointment with the dermatologist to see what new medications might improve the acne-like rosacea I had been resigned to suffer with for seven long years.

And then the hand of God stepped in once more, and I came face to face with the realities of what so many years of abusive overeating had done to the skin all over my body. I scheduled a consultation with a cosmetic surgeon.

Tummy tuck information overload

I hadn't planned on visiting a cosmetic surgeon during my retreat in Idaho. It just happened. Only I don't believe things "just happen." I believe there is always a reason, a purpose, a destiny.

I'd gone into a fitness center to check on the availability of a recumbent bike. Although only days out of my cast, I'd been able to ride such a bike throughout my heel immobility, and I knew I needed to get back on track with my exercise program. Unfortunately, the center had no such apparatus, and regular bikes, with their more vertical set-ups, adversely affected my knee joints.

As I returned to my car, I noticed the other businesses sharing the building. The office door of a cosmetic surgeon was adjacent to where I'd parked. I stepped inside and came face to face with a wall of brochures.

"May I help you?" the receptionist asked.

"I'm looking for information on tummy tucks," I told

her. Just saying the words aloud knotted my stomach, my mouth went dry, and I felt instantly queasy.

She came out from behind the counter and selected four pamphlets from the racks. The first was on "Abdominoplasty," the second on "Liposuction," and the remaining two were profiles of the doctors sharing the office facilities.

"Why don't start by reading these?" she suggested. "Then if you're interested in more information, you can call and schedule a complimentary consultation."

"Complimentary? As in 'free'?"

"As in 'free', and 'no obligation whatsoever'." She smiled. "The office visit takes about an hour, and I have an opening tomorrow afternoon."

The following afternoon a very nice doctor talked to me for some time about my current self-image, expected changes in my self-concept after surgery, and the value of listening to Tony Robbins' motivational tapes. He showed me a three-ring notebook containing before and after pictures of other clients, thoroughly answered most of the questions on my lengthy list, and then asked me to disrobe.

I stood in front of a large mirror, wearing nothing but a triangle-shaped, postage-stamp bikini bottom with strings. He used a word I had not read in the brochures. It started with "circum-something" and I figured it derived from the word circumference. He showed me where the incision would begin, back near my spine, and how it would progress around my hips and along my pelvis.

His assistant took notes and wrote down measurements while the doctor pressed his hands in around my hips, pulled and manipulated my massive abdominal flesh, gently but firmly grappling with the (*in my mind*) abhorrent amount of excess tissue hanging from my frame. He showed me what he would, and would not, be able to remove. Then, he said, he would make a cut higher on my "new" stomach area, and reinsert my navel.

I felt a tidal wave of nausea churning in my gut, so I nodded in supposed comprehension, but said nothing.

Next he had me hold my arms straight out from my sides and told me of two different options for dealing with the flapping masses of flesh hanging there. Basically, it amounted to either sucking the fat out and then pulling the skin up under my arm before cutting it off, or cutting from the elbow to the shoulder directly, leaving more of a scar.

After the arms, he said, we could tackle the thighs. The thighs were going to take a lot of work, he informed me, again pressing the skin around from the back and firmly grasping the flesh he would remove.

"And of course, you'll want your breasts lifted." He pinched the skin high on my chest and demonstrated where he felt my breasts *should* be. "I don't think you need any augmentation," he said, "but a good six to eight inch lift would make you feel like a whole new woman."

The nausea surged up into my throat. Once we started this nip and tuck process, would there be no end?

The doctor had me get dressed and then sat down with me to answer the last of my questions.

All in all, he suggested four major surgeries. The first one, which I still thought of as a 'tummy tuck,' would take five or six hours under general anesthetic. I'd be in the hospital four or five days. For two or three weeks afterward, there would be four shunts draining the fluid created by the swelling. I'd have to walk a little stooped over for a few weeks. Full recovery, provided there were no complications, would take four to six weeks. The cost was roughly $18,000 to $20,000 for this first procedure.

The arms could be done a month or so later, and cost another five or six grand. Then the thighs, ranging from eight to ten thousand, and for the breast lifting, another five or six thousand dollars.

I did the math. For $42,000, I could have back some semblance of the body I had before. And none of this was covered by insurance. None. Ruefully, I considered that I finally had some sort of tangible answer to the previously rhetorical question, "What was the cost of obesity?"

Forty-two thousand dollars, four major surgeries, a year or better for recovery, scars making jagged road maps across my entire body, and no guarantees I wouldn't die under anesthetic, which, given my medical history, was certainly a possibility.

"I'm not yet at my goal weight," I told him. "How long do you suggest I wait after I get to goal to see how much skin tightens up on its own?"

For a long moment, the doctor looked at me without comment. Then he blinked. "No need to wait at all," he said, gathering up his papers and clipping them inside my chart. "If you had lost this weight in your 30s, you would have 80% of your skin elasticity left, but you're 47. Your skin elasticity is zero. Just like a balloon that has been blown up too many times, the elasticity is gone. The reality is that your skin is just going to hang there. You have to decide if you can live with that, or if you're going to have it trimmed off. Remember what we discussed earlier about your self-concept? You've lost a lot of weight, and done a remarkable job of reclaiming your former life. What is the ultimate image you see for yourself?"

I contemplated his question. "What about those firming lotions containing vitamins A and E? Won't that help tighten the skin up *a little*?"

He smiled a small smile, then reached out and patted my knee in a rather condescending manner. "You call me when you're ready to schedule."

I nodded and stood to leave. By the time I got into my car, I was crying so hard I probably shouldn't have driven, but Steve's house was less than a mile away. I hobbled up the stairs to his home, went inside, threw myself across the bed, and bawled like there was no tomorrow.

I kept trying to tell myself it was only a little skin, and I was being irrational and somewhat silly. Nevertheless, depression settled over me like a heavy smothering blanket.

That's what friends are for

I couldn't shake it off. I paced back and forth through Steve's living room, and into the kitchen, opening and closing the refrigerator time and time again. My emotions ricocheted from indescribable pain to violent rage. *It just wasn't fair!* I'd come too far! Why was God throwing yet another obstacle in my path? Why couldn't I have my original body back?

Waist-deep into my pity-party, I felt myself sinking further and further down into the big black abyss of depression. And as I had always done when faced with such incredibly overwhelming feelings, my instant impulse was to grab as much comfort food as possible and quickly shove it into my mouth.

Six hundred fifty miles from home, I stood in Steve's bathroom and stared the reality of my massive quantities of epidermis square in the belly button. I was alone and isolated. No one would ever have to know if I succumbed to self-medicating with chocolate, or candy, or pastries, or ice cream, or anything and everything else I could get my hands on. The grocery store was close by, and it was a couple hours before Steve returned home. By then I could be happily numbed—zombied out in a sordid food coma.

But this time I didn't do it. This time, by the grace of God, I managed to use the tools advocated by my support group. I picked up the telephone instead.

I needed help and I needed it now, now, *now*, and right this very minute! I spent the next few hours telling my tale. I called Maggie, I called NY David, I called some of my friends back home, and every time I told my story, I gave a little more of the pain away. Granted, it still hurt like hell, but I was beginning to cope without resorting to stuffing my feelings down with food.

When Steve pulled into the driveway, we sat together on the couch, tears still rolling freely down my cheeks and dripping off my chin, and I told him about the trauma of my day. He quietly held my hand and let me talk until, at long last, I was all talked out.

"You don't have to decide anything today," he said softly.

I nodded.

"You can decide if you want the surgeries after you've been at goal a few months."

I nodded again.

"I know you probably thought when you lost all your weight that you'd have your former body back just like it was in high school."

Again I bobbed my head. Steve, like Maggie, and NY David, and the other support friends I had called during my desperate afternoon, had really heard me. They understood. They sympathized. They supported me unconditionally, no matter what I did or didn't decide to do.

There was only one more phone call to make. I had a sane dinner with Steve and got myself back under some semblance of emotional control before dialing my new gentleman friend's number.

I calmly summarized my dilemma to him. Six hours under anesthetic, drainage shunts, possibility of infections, abscesses, scars, and the appalling cost of just the first of four or five surgeries.

My new friend listened without much comment. I already knew he was looking for a smaller, leaner woman. I guess I expected him to tell me to go for the surgery or say good-bye, and I had prepared myself for that.

"It's up to you," he said. "Don't do it for me."

I knew he meant what he said. I also knew right then and there whether I ultimately chose to have some of my loose skin removed or not, he never said he would stay, and he never said he would go.

I made a conscious decision at that moment to remember all I needed to do was turn my relationship with this man over to the care of God. God's will, not mine. Only time would tell if this man would eventually accept me, "guts, warts, feathers and all."

Gratitude, gratitude, gratitude

I returned from my Idaho retreat a different person. Not the person I had expected to emerge from my three-week hiatus, but it was the one my Higher Power chose to send back home.

Whereas I thought I would be resolving some tough questions and issues concerning my emotional clarity, I came back to the beach with more unsettling distress than when I'd left. And of course, I wanted to eat over it.

Overeating had always been my favorite way of coping with unpleasant and uncomfortable feelings, and it was with white-knuckled determination I kept from returning to my old familiar pattern.

Depression over the sagging skin constantly plagued me, and I worked to accept with humility that there were some things I simply could not control. The first thing I decided was I didn't need to make a decision concerning "cosmetic" surgery until I was at goal weight for a few months, and *that* blessed event was still out on the horizon.

I reconnected with my friends in the support group and brought everyone up to speed concerning my revelations during my retreat. Many women in the group had been pondering similar questions about skin reduction, and although I tried to shut down my emotions and give "just the facts," my feelings were pretty raw. I cried again as I related my perceived humiliation and inadequacy.

After the meeting, one of the women took me aside and asked if I had read Christopher Reeve's book "Still Me." I had not. "You should read it," she said. "I bet he'd be happy to have his worst problem be a little sagging skin."

"It's not *a little sagging skin*," I replied, lifting my shirt to squeeze my bare midsection and show her just how much flab was hanging off me.

"You missed my point," she said softly.

I put the brakes on my self-pitying tirade long enough to focus on what she said.

"Every day Christopher Reeve has to have someone massage his abdomen with their fist just so he can have a bowel movement."

I remained silent.

"How do you think that makes him feel?" she asked

rhetorically. "Don't you think he wishes it were otherwise? Don't you think he wants his former life back? Don't you think he feels incredibly humbled at what he must submit himself to every single day *just to have a freaking bowel movement?!*" She paused for her words to sink in.

"Yet Christopher Reeve is glad to be alive, grateful that he's who he is, counts his blessings, and is unwilling to sink into the 'poor me' abyss."

"So you think I should be grateful for this abundance of loose, flabby skin?"

"I think you'd do well to put it in perspective, and take time every day to list your gratitudes."

"My gratitudes?" I thought for a minute. "You mean something like the fact I have released so much life-threatening weight that I *have* this much skin hanging?"

"Yeah," she said, "something like that. And while you're at it, you could start looking at your stretch marks as nothing more than battle scars, and your sagging skin as a badge of courage, a true testimony to distance you have worked so hard to come."

I gave my friend a long, heart-felt hug, and drove home from the meeting with a sense of awe that God had slowed me down long enough to get this message. I determined to make more of an effort to lean towards the optimism in each new day, and to find more ways to be grateful for what *is*, rather than irrationally despondent over what *isn't*.

But it's progress, not perfection, and I also instinctively knew this was a lesson I might have to repeat on a regular basis. Whether the glass is half full or half empty is a conscious choice, and I'm grateful I have true friends who will remind me of that as need be.

Incremental friends

With the convenience, and the mixed blessings, of telephone answering machines, voice mail, email, etc., many of the people I called my friends saw me face-to-face only on rare occasions.

One such occasion occurred the first Saturday of July, 2001. The local bookstore hosted an annual authors' party and/or book signing with 15 or 20 writers in attendance. I felt honored to be included, to date having had just one "real" book published—a collection of newspaper columns I'd written long before I began caring about my weight.

I arrived a few minutes before the appointed time and saw I would be sharing a table with Dr. Robert Michael Pyle, one of my author heroes. I'd known Bob for years, and had shared many a laugh and good story with him.

I approached our designated space and saw him setting up his impressive book display. I enthusiastically greeted him. "Dr. Pyle! How good to see you!"

Bob turned and stuck out his hand. "Bob Pyle," he said, "and your name?"

I thought he was kidding with me. "What's with the handshake crap?" I asked, grinning and opening my arms wide. "We've been hugging way too long to go back to shaking hands now!"

Bob's face went through a whole series of expressions in just a few seconds. First he looked genuinely puzzled, then shocked, and as the realization finally settled in, more than a little chagrined. "*Oh my God!*" he exclaimed, wildly gesturing with both arms to all the others to gather around. "*Has everyone seen Jan?*"

Some had, some hadn't. "I recognized the voice," said one writer, "but the body's sure not what I remember."

"I was blindsided," admitted another. "It's been two years since I've attended this gathering. What a difference two years makes!"

One writer acquaintance shook her head and laughed as she said, "I was just about to ask you if you had a sister named Jan. How embarrassing would *that* have been?"

Writer friends who were in more frequent direct contact with me stood nearby, beaming as if they had been on the inside of a really fine secret. These were my "incremental friends," who had witnessed the stages of my metamorphosis as it transpired.

My boyfriend *(and I used that term loosely),* settled into the chair meant for me and watched as I circulated throughout the room. I was mindful that he was more than a little uncomfortable, and strove to put him at ease by introducing him to a couple people there I thought he could talk to for a few minutes while I said my hellos.

But all anyone wanted to chat about was my miraculous transformation. Up until then, I don't think the magnitude of my change had hit home with my gentleman friend. He'd never seen me at the apex of my size. He had not even seen pictures of me as I had been then. He knew the numbers, but for him to experience these people's reactions was something neither one of us had expected when I invited him to attend the soiree.

He listened as the writers I would like to call my colleagues spouted their love and support, and there he sat, all too aware, I'm sure, of the fact I was receiving unconditional acceptance from them, but not yet from him. He still had "issues" with my weight, he had told me so only a couple hours before, and I couldn't help but wonder whether those "issues" would ever be totally resolved.

Shoving those thoughts into the back of my mind for

the time being, I allowed myself to bask in the limelight of my infamy, or perhaps small (*calorie-free*) potatoes notoriety, and thoroughly enjoyed the attention. I had, after all, earned every minute of it.

Willing to go to any lengths

I often marvel at the extremes I went to in order to gain and maintain my almost 400 pound weight for such a long period of time. While I didn't exactly set my alarm clock to get up in the middle of the night in order to eat additional calorie-laden food, it took quite a bit of fortitude, as well as planning, to ingest four to six thousand calories every 24 hours, day in and day out, for over a decade.

One of my moments of greatest insanity took place while standing at the counter of the local McDonald's. "I'd like two Happy Meals," I began. "One with orange juice and one with a diet cola." Then I stood there and pretended to scrutinize the menu above the server's head, as if I didn't have it memorized.

"And we need one super-sized extra value meal number three. Put a large chocolate milkshake with that." I hesitated again. "And for me," I lied through my teeth, "I'll just have a grilled chicken sandwich, no mayo, and a diet pop. Oh, and since those fruit pies are still two for a dollar you better throw some in. Make it four pies; the kids love them."

Did I really fool anyone? I sure thought I did. "And the Oscar for best obsessive/compulsive out-of-control overeater goes to..." But any dolt with fairly reasonable eyesight could take one look at me and see that I did not subsist solely on grilled chicken sandwiches sans mayo.

If anyone had followed me to my car as I left the fast-food restaurant, they would have seen me stuffing a fistful of fries into my mouth even before I got out of the parking lot. From there, I usually drove straight to the nearest beach approach and turned the front seat of my car into a virtual smorgasbord. The car's CD player provided dinner music; the ocean provided a view almost as vast as my waistline.

I laughed as the foolish seagulls clustered around my car, their keen eyesight obviously discerning a big red and yellow "M" on the paper food bags. No way were they getting even one measly French fry from me! I *needed* to eat every single one of them. I'd probably waste completely away if I didn't gobble up every morsel of what I'd bought. And no way was I going to *pay* for food to throw to some mangy scavenger birds!

Now, of course, I wish that I *had* fed the fries to the seagulls, and everything else, too.

My refrigerator and cupboards were always bulging because I had perfected the talent of shopping at several different grocery stores every week, pretending I was stocking up on everything in their sale ad and would not be shopping anywhere else for another week or two.

What a life I'd been living! What lies I told myself and others! Here I was willing to go to all these lengths to assure myself of hanging on to an extremely unhealthy weight, but I didn't love myself enough at this juncture to stop the insanity. Oh, I'd previously given much lip-service to getting my food under control, but this was the first time I became willing to give up these destructive behaviors.

Almost a full two years into my recovery from compulsive overeating, I was still asking myself if I had completely surrendered the thought of ever taking the weight back. Was I willing to be sane about food for the rest of my life? Was I willing to honestly commit myself to saying I would *never* go back to my former craziness?

Was I willing to exercise more? Was I willing to pay several months in advance at my gym?

Was I willing to get rid of my "larger size" clothing? Or was I hanging onto it "just in case" I went back into the Twilight Zone of unlimited food? I rationalized that planning a garage sale took too much time to organize and I kept putting it off. So what was *that* all about? Was I hedging my bets by keeping my fat clothes handy?

Was I *truly* willing to go to any length to rid myself, once and for all, of this compulsion to overeat? Well, I thought so. I was traveling on the right road—of that I was sure. But could I leave the sanctuary of my familiar surroundings and venture out "on vacation?"

My gentleman friend had called to suggest a change in venue; some neutral turf where we would have no former relationship skeletons in the closet and where we could get to know each other better.

I wanted to accept the invitation, yet fat never takes a vacation, I reminded myself. I wondered if maybe my compulsion would look the other way while I took this mini-holiday to Las Vegas with my gentleman friend. It was my first experience traveling with a "normal" eater, and I faced the prospect with more than a little trepidation.

I realized sooner or later I was going to find myself in unfamiliar surroundings with unfamiliar food choices. I got down on my knees and prayed I was not setting myself up for ultimate failure.

For the first time in my life, I acknowledged to my support group buddy it was my faith in God that brought me to my knees, not my fear of the food. Feeling fully centered, I agreed to spend four days in the land of the endless buffets.

Las Vegas land mines

There are all kinds of roller coasters: emotional, metaphorical, and literal, just to name a few. When my gentleman friend called to invite me to vacation with him in Las Vegas, I managed to experience every one of those roller coasters in very short order.

My first free-fall came when I realized that in 105-degree weather, I wasn't going to get away with wearing long pants and long-sleeved blouses the whole time.

But I hadn't owned a pair of shorts in several decades. I'd also need a new swimsuit. *A swimsuit*? How could I dare put on a swimsuit and be seen in it by someone who made no bones about the fact he didn't like the way my body looked when fully dressed?

Never mind, I told myself, just be who you are. He invited you on this trip because he enjoys your company. Just relax and go with the flow.

Easier said than done, but I made the best of it. It was a good reason to go out and buy some modest knee-length jeans and a decent bathing suit. I have never liked to shop, but now I was delighted to discover I could buy things off the regular-sized racks, and that justified purchasing five times the clothes I needed for a four-day vacation.

Then there was the food issue. Food is relatively cheap in Las Vegas, and there's a buffet in every corner of every casino. Plan ahead, I told myself, and knowing my friend rarely eats breakfast, I packed a canned diet shake for each morning of our stay. While he might function just fine playing Russian Roulette with his blood sugar, I knew myself well enough to know I needed to eat sensible food throughout the day to avoid the emotional peaks and valleys that come with getting too hungry between meals.

What I hadn't planned on was that he would forego lunch and opt for a large slab of white chocolate raspberry cheesecake instead. White chocolate raspberry cheesecake just happens to be the very taste I want in my mouth when it's my time to die. It's a taste truly to die for, except I knew that just such a taste might also kill my resolve.

And although I *knew* this, I caved in and ate a goodly portion of the cheesecake he ordered. And he knew I would; he ordered it with two forks. *How can he want me thinner*, I asked myself, *and want me to share his dessert, too?* There were definitely some mixed signals here, and I didn't know what to make of any of them.

The worst-case scenario was I had attracted yet another type of food plan saboteur. I tried detaching myself from those thoughts and enjoy the vacation. By careful adherence to my own self-care, I knew I didn't have to be suckered into overeating. Later there would be plenty of time to figure out what kind of a partner I'd settled for this time—and what to do about it.

My next hurdle was an actual roller coaster. My friend loved them, and I used to love them too, but that seemed like an eternity ago. I hadn't been on a roller coaster in 23 years. When I had had other opportunities to go on these rides the previous two decades, I'd been afraid I was too large to fit in the seats, and had passed on the experience.

Now I had to decide if I was still the thrill seeker I'd been in my 20s, or if that part of me was gone forever. It took some incredible self-talk, a.k.a. "self-bullying," but I eventually experienced not only the New York, New York, Casino's "Manhattan Express" coaster with its 360-degree loop and heart-stopping barrel roll, but also the dizzying height of the Stratosphere's "Let It Ride High Roller" coaster, traversing the outside of the top of the tower, a full

909 feet above the ground. The adrenalin rush was well worth the wait.

The Folies Bergere presented a whole 'nother kind of challenge. Watching sequin-bedecked, ostrich-plumed young women strut their stuff across the stage filled me with such envy it required a tremendous amount of intestinal fortitude to stay seated for the entire show. Realizing I would never again be able to have the body I coveted sent my emotions roiling dangerously.

But I didn't have to eat over it. Acceptance was the answer. To accept the things I cannot change is truly an enlightened gift, and I amazingly got that gift wrapped up in neon while navigating the land mines of Las Vegas.

I am grateful I set my insecurities aside and went on that trip. My friend and I and came home from our travels with a better understanding of our similarities and respect for our differences. All in all, it was good to spend some time together "on neutral ground," though it became clear in the weeks ahead that his image of "the perfect woman" couldn't be modified after all.

Soon, I had to accept the fact that I was unable to teach him good people come in all sizes, and forced to send him packing. Once again, my life literally depended on it.

CHAPTER VII:
FIRST DOWN AND GOAL TO GO

Super-sized garage sale

By the time I returned from Las Vegas I was finally, *finally!* ready to part with some of my larger-sized clothing.

I had been shifting clothes from one closet to another for almost two years, hesitant to commit myself to the idea that *this time* I wasn't going to take the weight back. I was actually afraid to get rid of them—afraid what I saw in the mirror wasn't there to stay.

But after thoroughly examining my vacation photos, and *trusting* what I saw was who I was now, I realized a garage sale was long overdue. I placed a newspaper ad.

"*LARGE WOMEN'S CLOTHING SALE.* Over 300 excellent condition blouses, dresses, pants and more. Many still with store tags attached! Sizes 40 to 60, XL to 6X, and 18 to 24. One day only."

"Over 300 items?" asked my friend Judy, helping me prepare for the sale. "Who in the world has over 300 items of new or gently used clothing they want to part with?"

"Some of them were purchased simply because when I found clothing that covered a 396 pound body, I grabbed it," I explained. "I used to buy 'one of every color and print' from mail-order catalogs that carried size 60, or 6X. Other clothes were 'transitional' as I worked my way back down the scale. I'm just lightening the load, and getting rid of the things that are definitely too big."

The day of the sale, Judy manned the cash box while I flitted among the shoppers. A strange sense of mourning overtook me as I watched armloads of clothing leave the garage. At first I didn't know exactly *why* I felt so sad, but I acknowledged and honored the grief as it washed over me.

Was there such a thing as post-partum blues over clothing? While I was delighted to be ridding myself of so many things I no longer needed, I still experienced a genuine sense of loss.

One woman was absolutely thrilled to find some "better" dresses in larger sizes that she could wear to work. As she removed my all-time favorite dress from the hanger, I put my hand gently over hers.

"Promise me you're going to give that dress a good home," I said. I couldn't believe the catch in my throat.

She smiled. "I take it there's a lot of history leaving here today?"

"That's the dress I wore when I danced barefoot on the beach under a full moon one night a couple years ago. The sand that clung to the hem the next day reminded me of stardust. The guy I danced with is long gone, and when this dress leaves with you today, all I'll have left is a distant memory and a poem I wrote about it."

"I understand," she said quietly. "Thanks for sharing that story with me."

As I circulated throughout the garage, many women asked me what I'd done to lose so much weight. I had anticipated this curiosity, and had practiced a few glib responses to avoid getting into long conversations during the prime sale time: "I stopped eating so much." "I sewed my mouth shut." "I gave up food for lent one year, and forgot to take it back up after Easter."

I really didn't mind their questions, and for a sincere few, I slowed down long enough to talk seriously with them for a couple minutes.

"You've been following a food plan for over *two years?!*" said an incredulous woman. "I don't know if I'll even be *alive* two years from now!"

I held her gaze for a moment before responding. "There's a pretty good chance you'll live longer if you commit yourself to a lifetime food plan today. Are you ready to make that commitment to yourself?"

"It's not a good time right now," she hastily replied. "I'm going on vacation next week, and then there's the family reunion, and my daughter is coming to visit next month, and my husband won't eat what I eat if I start trying to eat healthy and..."

I excused myself to go help another customer.

The nature of my newspaper ad, as well as the signs I posted along the roadways, discouraged most men from walking up the driveway. Big bold letters advertising a "Large Women's Clothing Sale" encouraged most of them to drive on by. But one man ventured in anyway, accompanying his wife. Hands in pockets, he took a cursory look around and then asked in a loud, booming voice, "Where's the fat lady?"

My stomach instantly knotted. I was barely able to keep from saying what I was thinking. This man was obviously a total jerk. I pitied his wife, a large woman who now had a very red face, timidly walking a few steps behind him. I turned away and continued to bite my tongue.

"Hey," he repeated in an even louder and more obnoxious tone, "I asked where the fat lady was."

"The fat lady," I replied, forcing my voice to remain

calm, "doesn't live here anymore. And unless you're going to allow these women to continue shopping without any more of your verbal abuse, I'll have to ask you to leave."

The man turned on his heel and abruptly left the property. His wife looked at me with such pain in her eyes that I saw a startling glimpse of the hell she must have endured each day. I said a silent prayer for her as I watched her walk away empty-handed, her shoulders decidedly stooped. There are worse things than being alone, I reminded myself.

For the most part, the sale was a win-win situation. Larger women in my area had few opportunities to get quality clothing at reasonable prices, and I was only too happy to capitalize on that fact. I'd put price tags of five or 10 dollars on most of the nicer blouses, which is a little high for normal garage sales, but very few haggled prices. I told them the numbers were firm for the day, but I'd be having a one hour half price sale on Sunday if they thought the item they wanted might still be there. No one was willing to take the chance.

By the end of the day, my sale had far exceeded my monetary imagination. After deducting the "change" Judy started with, I made out a deposit slip for $1,015, and all from clothing that no longer served me.

It was, as Martha Stewart often said, "a very good thing, indeed."

The last 10 to 30 pounds are the hardest

On the first of August, 2001, buck-naked clear down to my plum fingernail polish, I weighed an honest 179 pounds. This event brought an interesting question to the forefront. What *was* my ultimate weight "goal?"

When I began this odyssey, at 396 pounds, I had many incremental numerical goals. "Under 300" was mandatory. "Under 235," and I knew I would leave morbidly obese behind, and progress to simply being "very overweight." I determined at the onset I could live with that, presumably forever. From where I started, to be "under 200" was an impossible dream—a fantasy I only hoped to someday see.

But my ultimate "goal?" Back at 396, I looked longingly at my high school letter sweater, and at my wedding pictures, and at the size 14 and 16 clothes hidden deep in the back of my closet. I remembered with incredible tactile sense clarity what it felt like to be between 168 and 178. And I desperately wanted to feel that way again.

So I had set my "sugar-free pie in the sky" goal at anywhere between 168 and 178. And here I was, August 1, 2001, at 179. And I knew in my heart, as well as by looking in the mirror, that another 2 to 12 pounds wasn't going to be quite enough to satisfy me.

It being the first of the month, I took my various body measurements and dutifully recorded them on my progress chart. Those numbers weren't quite enough either.

How much more was it reasonable to want to lose? The plenitude of loose, hanging skin was making it difficult to see my true shape underneath. The cosmetic surgeon had said the skin weighed only 5 to 8 pounds, but poundage aside, it was now definitely in the way of my fitting into a size or two smaller clothing.

What part was vanity starting to play? I looked pretty good in size 12 pants and size 14 to 16 tops, as long as they were long-sleeved. The "angel wings," as my friend Miki called them, were driving me crazy. I hated the way I felt when they wiggled and jiggled, and consciously tried to keep from writing on the blackboard or putting my hands in the air in front of anyone. I didn't *want* to feel I had to spend the rest of my life in long sleeves, but surgery was rapidly becoming the only viable option to avoid that.

I would not consider skin-reduction surgery until I reached "goal," I kept telling myself, yet I was still unable to define my ultimate "goal."

I began scrutinizing other women approximately my height, trying to decide if I was heavier or thinner than they were. As if my "worth" were determined by relative size! That was clearly stinkin' thinkin', and as soon as I acknowledged what I was doing, I turned my eyes inward and prayed for serenity to come at any number on the scale.

My quasi-boyfriend suggested I "shoot for 130 to 135." When he told me that, I wanted to shoot *him*. "This isn't *your* goal for me," I reminded him, "it's *my* goal for me. And I think 158 to 168 just might be perfect."

As soon as the numbers came out of my mouth, I knew them to be true. To lose another 10 to 20 pounds seemed exceptionally reasonable, and then I could tackle the exciting, and difficult adventure of "maintenance."

The very idea of maintenance scared me. I was pretty good at *losing* weight, and I was obviously very good at *gaining* weight, but to maintain one constant weight "forever" seemed like another one of my pipe dreams.

So I spent the month of August yo-yoing a few pounds here and there, and by the first of September had dropped only two and a half pounds. Well, two and a half pounds is still two and a half pounds, and I was grateful I hadn't had a net gain. But it didn't bring me all that much closer to my "goal." So why was I dragging my feet?

Perhaps it was my fear of maintenance that kept me from working harder on my physical recovery. All I knew for sure was at this rate, it could be 8 to 10 months before I had to face that maintenance hurdle, and suddenly 8 to 10 more months wasn't going to cut it.

It was time to kick it up a notch. I added more time at the gym and more walks to my schedule. I didn't really think I could trim too many more calories from my daily intake and still function, but additional exercise always made me feel better for having done it. A rush came with the idea of those little endorphins running around with little serotonin cocktails that invigorated me.

Looming not very far out there on the horizon was the "Great Columbia Crossing," the 6.2 mile "Bridge Walk" that my heel spur had kept me from the previous year. It was time to start training in earnest for my next big challenge. And I do mean *big*.

Maggie and Miki yet again

School began a few days before Labor Day. And although I'd be lying if I didn't admit I'd much rather spend my days doing the things I had time to do during summer, the structure of being back at work put additional discipline into my ability to stick to a food and exercise plan.

Maggie and Miki and I were all teachers. Maggie taught elementary music, Miki taught in the primary grades, and I worked with junior high and high school students.

Although our assignments varied, in September, 2001, Maggie and Miki and I returned to our classrooms with something rather spectacular in common. We went back to work with our weights hovering just above 170—nothing short of a miracle.

Collectively, by this date the three of us had released

somewhere in the vicinity of 470 pounds over the past 2 1/2 years. Four hundred seventy pounds! Unfathomable!

But none of the three of us were yet "at goal." Our goal weights were so tantalizingly close, but not one of us could honestly say it was time to begin the maintenance phase of our journeys.

The closer I got to goal, the harder it was to stay the course. My obsession with food overtook most other waking thoughts. As soon as I got up in the morning, I started thinking about what I could eat for breakfast. Before breakfast was over, I had a begrudgingly light lunch all planned. By the time school got out in the late afternoon, I'd already be counting the minutes till I could inhale a somewhat substantial dinner.

I began to wonder what "normal" people thought about all day. "Lunch is coming," I told myself throughout the morning as my hunger pangs clamored for attention. "Dinner's coming," was my standard afternoon mantra.

My "lifetime food plan" was threatening to turn into a "diet." And, as I'd said so many times before, "If you go *on* a diet, then you will eventually go *off* a diet." Unless I wanted to reclaim my weight, plus some, I couldn't afford to be thinking like that.

Maggie and Miki were also finding it difficult to break through their own individual plateaus. It seemed we three had "hit the wall," and the wall wasn't giving an inch. I knew in my heart I had slacked off on my daily vigilance and I could ill afford to run even a little bit fast and loose with my food plan. Writing down every single thing I ate was vital, and yet days passed where I'd been less than honest or too lazy to record it.

My solution was to turn my attention to what had worked best for me thus far. In addition to beefing up my exercise plan of gym time and daily walks, I started attending more support group meetings. "Misery loves company," I told myself.

It took me awhile to admit attending meetings wasn't "misery" at all, but a time of joyful fellowship. And besides, just being at a meeting kept me away from the fridge for an hour or two, and that in itself was time well spent.

Time and time again at those meetings I heard "Compulsive eating is a disease that wants you dead." I let the idea totally soak in. As with any addiction, the key to recovery is to take it one day at a time, to admit you are powerless over it, and to turn it over to a Higher Power.

"Okay, H.P.," I said aloud as I drove home from a meeting one evening. "I surrender this little problem of mine completely to you. You can have it!"

Thankfully, God was listening. I got back on track, and had a few blessedly abstinent days strung together before the world, as we knew it, was forever changed.

9/11—Sugar won't fix it

On September 11, 2001, at exactly 6:15 a.m. Pacific Daylight Time, I entered a small local convenience store to pick up a cup of coffee on my way to an early morning faculty meeting.

Several men stood clustered together beneath a wall-mounted television set just inside the door. They were staring up at the screen, and no one was saying a word. I could tell by the looks on their faces something horrible was being projected above their heads. I also knew in my gut I didn't want to know what it was that had their attention so intently riveted.

September 11, 2001. A day in which we saw, with all too much clarity, the high level of American vulnerability. Our country had been attacked. *We* had been attacked. None of us would ever feel as safe again as we had when we'd gone to bed the night before.

I stood beside the men in silence. With a growing lump in my throat, nausea welling up in my stomach and tears blurring my vision, I gathered some form of small comfort standing there among the delivery truck drivers, the storeowner and a few early morning regular customers. It was not a time to be alone.

Soon, however, I realized I had a job to go to, and tore myself away from the repeated views of the unimaginable destruction on the television screen.

Our school staff functioned that day on a type of "automatic pilot." We talked in hushed tones as we wondered, and worried, about what to tell our students. We abandoned our lesson plans, and did our best to answer their questions as honestly and accurately as we could. But how do you explain the unexplainable? How do you reassure them everything will be all right when you're really not sure yourself it will *ever* be right again?

My 17 and 18-year-old students wanted to go sign up for military duty and blast anyone who lived on Middle Eastern sand to kingdom come.

"All Germans were not Nazis," I reminded them. "And all Muslims are not terrorists."

By noon, all I wanted to do was comfort myself with food. Lots and lots of food. Fear for the future, both my own future and the future of my students, pushed me hard to resort to prior food comforts. I wanted desperately to stuff down those feelings of fear and powerlessness. Those "eat until you can't eat another bite" pain-numbing strategies that had never served me well in the past were nevertheless pressing my panic buttons.

And I wanted to press some buttons back. During the lunch break I became fixated on the rows upon rows of candy and cookies and chips in the faculty room vending machine. I wanted to press the C-7 buttons until there weren't any more packages of M&Ms left leering at me.

"You know what I want?" asked one staff member aloud to no one in particular. "I want a drink. Make that a *lot* of drinks. I want to drink myself into a total stupor and wake up tomorrow and find out none of this happened–that it was all just a bad nightmare." He sighed heavily. "The hangover would be worth it."

Many of the faculty present nodded in whole-hearted agreement and expressed their preferences for a wide variety of alcoholic beverages.

I knew the man who had spoken quite well. I knew he had not had a drink in many years. I was relatively certain he would not be drinking that night either, and it floored me when he said he wanted to get shit-faced drunk. Yet I'd be the first to admit old, outdated coping skills die hard.

Why then, I wondered, did I think a quick "sugar fix" would make anything in *my* life better than if this man got drunk? Oh, it "sounded good," on the surface, but deep in my heart I knew eating several dozen candy bars would *not* restore the World Trade Center.

I tried rationalizing if war was imminent, and we were going to die anyway, that I might as well die with the taste of M&M peanuts in my mouth. What difference would it make if I died a few pounds heavier? All I wanted was chocolate. Oh, how I wanted chocolate! I wanted it like I had rarely wanted anything in my entire life.

But I didn't have it.

What stopped me? I honestly don't know. Divine Intervention, perhaps. I had enough change in my purse to buy out every package of M&Ms, both peanut *and* plain, as well as several other types of predominantly chocolate candy in the machine. But I didn't do it.

I chalk it up to God's grace. God knew I had to be at the top of my form to help my students get a handle on what was happening in their world. And God knew I couldn't do that if I was in a freaked-out highly dysfunctional sugar coma. My kids, then and always, came first.

T minus 7 and counting

The Great Columbia Crossing was about to happen, whether I was ready or not. Was I ready? My goal, ever since I had the bone spur removed from my heel in mid-March, was to have the ability to walk across the Megler/Astoria Bridge in October.

In the beginning, the doctor had told me it would be six to nine months before I had "full recovery." Later he amended it to "nine to twelve months." But that was until I could reasonably expect to be "pain free." What's a little pain, I rationalized, if I can accomplish my goal and be none the worse for wear? The date of the Bridge Walk was six months and two weeks after my heel had been cut open.

With only seven days before the scheduled walk, I was having my doubts. For three consecutive days my foot had been feeling like I wasn't going *anywhere* the weekend after next, much less walking the bridge.

But early on the last Sunday in September I awoke with a sense of complete bliss and inner peace. First daylight filtered into my bedroom and I lay there watching the colors come alive outside my window. I could tell it was going to be a gorgeous early autumn morning.

I took inventory of my body. Nothing in particular seemed to be hurting—a good sign. I rolled out of bed about 7 a.m. and pulled on my gym clothes. I strapped on the fanny pack a normal-sized friend had lent me for the Bridge Walk and discovered, much to my amazement, I didn't have to adjust the waistband! I did a couple warm-up stretches, leaning against the wall and manipulating my leg muscles. No doubt about it, I felt *good*.

I left my house and headed north along the roadway into a considerable wind coming directly at me. Best to walk into the wind on the trip out, I told myself, so I could take advantage of a tailwind coming back.

When I had gone a little over a mile, I walked past a newly-cleared potential housing development. Two large deer, grazing in the clearing, abandoned their breakfast and accompanied me for quite some distance. They kept pace with me, just on the other side of the roadside brush and a formidable ditch, following along like a couple large and well-trained dogs.

I climbed a short, curved incline on the road to my usual "turnaround" driveway, but decided to push the envelope and walk a little farther.

When I finally headed for home, I knew I'd be completing a few tenths over 3 miles when I got back to my own driveway. But when I actually got there, my little voice said, "You can do it—keep walking." So I did. I walked another six or seven tenths of a mile south before I turned.

Naturally, I hopped in the car as soon as I got home and set the trip odometer on zero. I drove the route I had just walked and was delighted to discover it was a full 4.6 miles! And I *knew*, right then and there, with all the faith of absolute certainty, if the Bridge Walk had been that morning, I could have done the full 6.2 miles—the full 10K. I was completely confident I could walk a little less than another 2 miles without problem. And that fact in itself was something to celebrate.

Whether or not I was able walk the full Bridge Walk the following weekend was suddenly irrelevant, on *that particular day*, I *knew* I could have done it!

It had taken me one hour and 23 minutes to walk 4.6 miles. That left 37 minutes of my two-hour maximum Bridge Walk time limit to walk the final 1.8. It was definitely "doable," even though there *was* that "challenging incline" on the south end of the bridge.

But maybe all I really needed to know was I "could have" done it. The distance that I'd come, both literal and metaphorical during the past two years, had been nothing short of awe-inspiring. And I knew, deep in my heart of hearts, confronting the bridge itself was almost after the fact. *Almost.*

I was as ready for this odyssey as I was ever going to be. Whether I finished the walk or got picked up by the "sweeper bus," I knew I was going to be okay with it, because on this particularly beautiful Sunday morning I felt like the little engine who knew she could.

A long and arduous journey

On Sunday, October 10, 1999, my friend New York David had challenged me to define my long-term goals. "Dare to dream big," he told me. "In your wildest imagination, what would you like to see?"

I had thought for a long moment before replying. "I

want to be healthy. I want to lose a significant amount of weight. I want to be active and fit. I want to go dancing with you in a red sequined dress."

"Is that it?"

"And," back then I had taken a deep breath, "today's the Great Columbia Crossing, otherwise known as The Bridge Walk. It's 10 kilometers, which is 6.2 miles. In my wildest imagination, I want to do The Bridge Walk."

"Why?"

"Why? What kind of a question is 'why'?"

"Why is this important enough to put on your list of goals? You must have a reason," he said.

I *did* have a reason, and not a very pretty one. A couple years before, a friend and I were out walking on some Leadbetter Point State Park trails and we had gotten the signs confused. We walked a mile or two in the wrong direction before we discovered our mistake, and had to turn around and walk the same dune trail all the way back.

It was 80-something degrees at the time, we had no water with us, no hats to keep off the sun, and I was more than 200 pounds overweight. Before we arrived back at the parking lot, I nearly collapsed twice. My friend had suggested going on alone and calling for medical assistance for me from the parking lot, but I had struggled on. My face turned deep purple, and as I gasped for air, I felt certain that heat stroke, and perhaps even death, was imminent.

I swore at the time that by the following year I would be able to trot right along those trails, but by the following year my weight had climbed even higher. I was no longer in contact with my friend, so I rationalized that there was no need to go walking those dune trails ever again.

But although my weight-loss efforts for several years had been less than whole-hearted attempts, I never lost the desire to someday be able to walk where and when I wanted to walk.

I tried to explain all this on the phone.

New York David had listened attentively. "How far are you able to walk right now?" he had asked.

"Honestly?"

"Honestly."

"I have to rest between the car and the house."

NY David didn't hesitate. "Then go for it," he had said. "I'll be rooting for you."

In 2000, my attempt at the Bridge Walk had been thwarted by a heel spur, but a year later, post-surgery, I was ready to try again.

I awoke on Sunday, October 7, 2001, at 3:08 a.m. (*The curse of digital clocks is knowing exactly what time sleep eludes you.*) I tossed and turned for over an hour, reciting over and over my practiced litany: "Defeat is not an option. Forward is the only viable direction. Hope springs eternal. I think I can, I think I can, I think I can..."

At 9 a.m. I stood at the starting line in the Megler Rest Area with over 2,000 others. An all-day coastal drizzle failed to dampen my spirits. I had two hours to cross the bridge or the "sweeper bus" would load me up with the rest of the stragglers. Six and almost a quarter miles, with a "challenging incline" near the five-mile mark.

But even before I took the first step, I knew beyond a shadow of a doubt I was already a winner. I had lost 220 pounds in two years. My cholesterol was 141, my resting blood pressure a mere 130/74.

In my borrowed fanny pack I carried various "tokens" as proudly as a medieval knight carried his beloved's handkerchief into the tournament games. I had 15 small metal "Angels of Hope" tucked in there, along with gum, breath mints, a disposable camera, a small rock with "Patience" written on it, another that said "Gratitude," and of course, my original marbled purple "Hope Rock." The angel-coins I planned to give away to others in my support group who were walking the bridge with me "in spirit."

On my rainbow-colored sweater I wore a button that said, "I'm having fun now!" and I was determined to keep that idea uppermost in my mind. I had shown up, suited up, and the outcome was not up to me. I was, I reminded myself one more time, already a winner.

My first mile clocked in at 14 minutes, 35 seconds. Amazing! At the end of the second mile my time was 31:30. The third mile registered 47 minutes and some-odd seconds. Then came the hill–six tenths of a mile with a steep uphill grade. Mile four was only a third of the way up the incline. Sixty-one minutes, 15 seconds.

I felt my resolve, along with my knees, begin to weaken. I didn't know if I could make it. I began walking slower and slower, my breathing becoming more labored as each second passed.

From among the throng surging ahead, a woman suddenly fell back and into step with me. She had curly long blonde hair and a cheery smile. "You can do it," she said. "I'll walk with you to the top."

She chatted merrily along as I struggled with each step. "I live on your side of the river," she told me. "I know who you are. I know you've lost a whole lot of weight. This walk is a big deal for you, isn't it?" I could only nod, tears threatening to mix with the still-falling drizzle.

God had sent me another angel, another Eskimo, to help me along. Right when I most needed confirmation of His love, this woman had appeared to hold my hand as I tackled the biggest physical challenge of my recovery. I thought, as my angel continued to talk, about the story of the "Footprints in the Sand," and how, when there were but one set of prints along the beach, that was when Jesus was carrying the load for His walking partner.

At the crest, I stopped long enough to throw my arms in the air while my angel snapped a picture reminiscent of Sylvester Stallone in "Rocky." I considered the enormity of my 220-pound release, and I imagined hefting 16 14-pound frozen turkeys up and over the side of the railing while screaming, "Fly, little birdies, fly!"

I felt totally happy, joyous, and free for the first time in over a decade. It felt good to be so giddy.

And then gravity took over. My feet flew out from under me. I whizzed by walker after walker. At mile five the clock keeper called out 77 minutes, and I became obsessed with finishing "in good time." I quickened my stride and gave that last mile and a quarter everything I had.

A couple hundred yards from the end, Michael, a former student of mine, appeared at my side. *Another angel?* I wondered, as he shouted his encouragement: "You can do it, Ms. B., you can do it!"

I smiled at him. "*Of course* I can do it!" I said. "Let's run!" And we ran the best I could, which wasn't pretty, but it was a little faster than my race-walking. I felt like I was galloping on bloody stumps instead of feet, but I kept going. The pain could wait.

As Michael and I approached the finish line together (*he had finished his actual race some 45 minutes ahead of me*), I threw my arms in the air for the second time and yelled to the crowd standing on both sides of the street, "Applause please! I'd like some applause!"

Loud clapping and raucous cheers greeted me as I soared across the finish line. My feet hardly touched the ground; I felt like I'd won the whole darn thing. The clock registered 1:34:15.

By the grace of God, and with the unfailing support of NY David and many, many others, I had done it—*we* had done it. Together we had done what I could never have done alone.

Somewhere along the route, the drizzle had turned to a steady rain. I collected my coveted "Great Columbia Crossing 10K Walk/Run" neck ribbon and medal, then headed for the car, where I had stashed a towel and a change of clothing.

As I unlocked the driver's side door, I looked up and over the top of my vehicle at the arch of the bridge in the distance. Many walkers still struggled with the incline on their own personal journeys. An enormous lump filled my throat and tears threatened once again.

"Thank you, God!" I called out in loud, clear voice. "Thank you, thank you, thank you!" And from all over the parking lot, I heard a chorus of other wet but happy runners and walkers calling out a hearty *"AMEN!"*

10/10 of 01

On the tenth day of the tenth month in the first year of the new millennium, I celebrated two full years of commitment to my food plan and program of recovery from compulsive overeating.

But once the Bridge Walk was over, once I'd reached the top of the hill, once I'd seen enough change in my appearance to start getting quite a bit of attention for my efforts, a funny thing happened. Not funny as in "ha-ha," but funny like in twisted, perverted, unsettling and discomfiting. At my time of greatest accomplishment, I began having my greatest doubts.

On the wall next to my desk was a quote that had been taped there for years. There was no attribution attached to it, and I couldn't remember the context in which it first struck my fancy. It said: "Something in human nature causes us to start slacking off at our moment of greatest accomplishment. As you become successful, you will need a great deal of self-discipline not to lose your sense of balance, humility, and commitment."

No kidding.

What they said in the support meetings was also true: If you rest on your laurels, your laurels will get bigger. I "should" have been feeling wonderful, but what I felt in my life was no euphoric joy, no real satisfaction.

I tail-spinned into a self-absorbed power slump. I felt I was living a two-year lie, like I was a fraud, and just faking it. I didn't feel any happier, and all my joints still hurt. Yet everyone looked at me like I was some kind of poster child for weight loss. I didn't want to be anyone's "hero." I just wanted to stay on my program and do the best I could, one day at a time.

I began having serious concerns (*and it was about time*), over my "relationships" with men who made me feel I would never be "good enough." What was I doing with men who thought I *chose* to overeat? Why had I settled for men who did not believe in the progressive compulsive nature of my disease, or even that I *had* a disease?

When I was with these guys, I felt shame and guilt. Instead of celebrating the success I'd had, I berated myself for not having more discipline, and less weight.

I needed my chosen "significant other" to be someone who was unconditionally supportive. My current so-called "boyfriend" hadn't even cared enough to be there when I completed the Bridge Walk. You call that support?

On the way to see him the following weekend, I began to sneak eat. I ate before I got to his house, then ate my regular dinner in front of him, then ate what I had squirreled away in my suitcase while he was out working in his shop. I couldn't eat in front of him; he'd be "watching." I had made him my "Food Police." I had given him an inordinate amount of power over me, and of course, I rebelled against it.

Every time I compulsively stuffed something into my mouth that weekend, I ran to the bathroom, or out behind the house, and tried to purge. I discovered, much to my misguided dismay, even by ramming my toothbrush half way down my throat, I could not induce vomiting. Damn! Damn! And double damn!

I cried nearly the whole weekend. My man friend thought it was PMS, or perhaps "the post Bridge Walk blues," and he suggested that once I set a new goal, I would get my volatile emotions back under control. But in my heart, I knew what the problem was, and simply didn't know if I was strong enough to fix it.

I went home at the end of the weekend knowing I would never see him again. It was time for me to eliminate some of the self-inflicted pain in my life. I had to save myself, but I knew what kind of emotional pain the breakup would cause. One more man in my life was about to be history. And once again, it would be by my own doing.

I wrote him a "Dear John" email. I had tried to tell him how I felt in person, but hadn't been able to look him in the eye and say good-bye. I tried to tell him on the phone, but he always twisted my words in ways that made me think I'd be nuts not to want him in my life.

So I sent him an email, and I never heard from him again. He didn't call, didn't come see me, didn't respond in any way, so naturally I figured I was right, and he hadn't cared that much to start with. I had often joked he needed a cocker spaniel for companionship more than he needed me. Perhaps I hadn't been joking after all.

I immediately became despondent and my weight started yo-yoing. This was my pattern of the past two years. Once again, I couldn't stick to my food plan for more than two consecutive days. I'd eat like crazy for two or three days, then gather some semblance of sanity and get back on track for another day or two. And the cycle repeated.

For over a month, I thought I could handle it, I thought I was "maintaining" and I prayed I wasn't headed for a massive relapse and inevitable weight gain.

Two arms! Two arms!

I reached up to write across the top of the blackboard and abruptly pulled my arm back down to my side. The three-quarter length sleeves on the blouse I was wearing had ridden up when I lifted my chalk-filled hand and the flabby skin hanging underneath noticeably flopped around like a salmon on a boat deck.

"Turn to page 178," I said to the language arts class, changing my lesson plan mid-stride. *How vain of me*, I thought, but how embarrassing, too.

The following day I went to a dress store in the Seaside outlet mall and discovered all their "summer" dresses were on clearance. I grabbed a handful in my approximate size and headed for the dressing room. Several of the dresses looked pretty good on me, but I left the store without buying anything. None of the dresses I'd tried on had sleeves long enough to disguise what I now referred to as "my disfigurement."

That afternoon I went online and began researching cosmetic surgeons within a 120-mile radius of my home. I found several, and started the arduous task of weeding through the salesmanship and propaganda to find what I thought might be "a good fit" between the doctor and/or clinic and myself.

Since the previous June, I had all but given up any idea of having the excess skin removed. The trauma of that initial consultation in Idaho had left considerable scar tissue on my psyche. But now my self-talk went into maximum overdrive.

This has nothing to do with my former gentleman friend, I reminded myself. It isn't vanity to want my body back in the approximate shape it had been in the last time I weighed this amount. It's about me feeling good about *me*. It's about self-esteem and wanting to be the best I can be. *Come on, girl—dig deep,* I told myself, *find the courage to change the things you can.*

During my first appointment at the clinic I eventually selected, I stood naked before the doctor and held my arms straight out from my sides once again. I twisted my wrists rapidly back and forth, causing the upper arm skin to wiggle and jiggle like Jell-O.

"Oh, I see you have bat wings," said the doctor.

"I prefer to call them *angel wings*," I informed her. "So how much will it cost if I just have my arms done?"

She checked the clipboard where she'd been making notations and said, "We can save you a lot of money if we combine procedures."

"How much is 'a lot'?"

"I think we can safely turn five surgeries into two," she replied.

My wheels began spinning in earnest as she explained—arms, abdomen, outer thighs first, then the inner thighs and lifting the breasts. Instead of a total of somewhere in the ballpark of $42,000, she was estimating the first surgery at around $15,000, and the second at $10,000. That suddenly sounded like one hell of a bargain.

But $25,000 was still $25,000, and I wondered where I'd get that kind of money. I wondered if Subway, where I'd been eating several times a week for over a year, would consider making me a Poster Child so I could finance these operations without going into bankruptcy.

I could get a new car for $25,000, I thought wryly. *OR,* said my ever-optimistic little voice, *you could get a whole new chassis.* A whole new chassis—I kind of liked that idea. A new chassis, or at the very least, a major tune-up or semi-complete overhaul.

I looked at my stomach in the full-length wall mirror and pressed the skin in from the sides. It puckered and bulged and looked a lot like I'd strapped a goose-fleshy 10 or 12 pound uncooked turkey to the front of my body. I thought longingly of my stomach lying flat once more; crisscrossed by stitches and road-mapped by bright-red scars, no doubt, but *without all this hanging flab.*

"I'm just a shade over five foot six inches," I slowly began. "I've been working out at the gym for an hour three times a week for almost a year. Underneath all this loose flesh I think I'm in pretty good shape. I weighed 176 this morning." I took a long breath. "Realistically, I probably need to lose another 15 or 20 pounds to be 'at goal'." I paused again. "So how long do you suggest I be at goal weight before the first surgery?"

The doctor took both hands and lifted one of the massive aprons of skin rolling down my belly and said, "The weight of the skin that will be removed will weigh somewhere between five and eight pounds. I think you're probably at your goal right now."

At goal?! Now? Not possible! *Or was it*?

I enjoyed a brief moment of elation, followed immediately by a petty little desire to have her put her assessment in writing so I could send a copy of this new information on to my former gentleman friend. I *am* at my goal weight! So there! Chew on *that*!

Fortunately, my temporary insanity passed quickly and I focused back on the moment at hand. I checked my school calendar. End of term, quarter grades due, my period due, spring break, state assessment testing, conferences. There didn't seem to be a particularly "good" time to do this. I teetered on the brink of chickening out.

The doctor sat with me in silence for a few minutes while I quietly collected my thoughts. It was late October. The holidays were coming, the roads might be icy in the winter, I had a lot of irons in the fire—but what about putting ME on the top of that to-do list?

"Ok," I said at last, "let's schedule it for March."

Licking the bottom of the brownie bowl

The very day I took the plunge and scheduled the long-awaited skin removal surgery, my commitment to eating sanely flew right out the window. I began hurriedly eating everything in sight, and then some. In my pea brain I rationalized I had two and a half years of "deprivation" to make up for and I determined to eat some of everything I had forgone all that time.

Naturally, this gorge-fest resulted in a total crash and burn. The fact I could trace the effect right back to the cause was no consolation.

The surgery scared me. Surgery has always scared me. There's something about being out of the driver's seat while under anesthetic makes me crazy. Or maybe that's "crazier." I worried about not waking up, not ever regaining consciousness, not living to tell the story. I worried after all the weight lost, I'd never enjoy the true fruits of my labors.

For 45 years, the way I coped with stress was to eat to numb the pain. If I had an "owie," a cookie would certainly make it better. Food was my constant safety net; if I hurt, eating would give me comfort. Now I planned on having weeks and weeks of "self-inflicted" pain, and there were four long months before the surgery date to worry about it. And to eat over it.

Somewhere between that first compulsive bite and the acknowledgment of once again being out of control and totally disregarding my food plan, I crossed the line from a slip to a full-blown relapse.

My car still knew, all too well, the way to the McDonald's drive-thru window. I could still wolf down a whole loaf of garlic bread while I waited for the water to boil to make enough spaghetti for a hungry family of six. A bag of tator tots was allegedly 11 servings of 180 calories each, but I could polish off the whole thing as a side dish. Leftover Halloween candy averaged 80 calories per piece, and I counted 60 wrappers as I cleared the evening's debris from the coffee table one night before bed.

I had gone from the top of the bridge to the valley of despair. Every night, tossing and turning, no doubt partially from acute indigestion, I had nightmares of weighing 396 pounds again. I felt like Humpty Dumpty, barely balanced on the ledge, several egg rolls short of sanity, yet I couldn't seem to derail the runaway the train.

The bottom line might be that success frightened me. At 170 I was about two pounds from my original goal. *Two pounds*! And yet, when it came right down to it, I think perhaps my stinking thinking was telling me if I filled all this loose hanging skin back up I wouldn't have to have the surgery at all.

Old habits die hard. It was obvious I couldn't do this alone, but I also couldn't find it within me to pick up the telephone and call for help. As I heard many times in my support group, compulsive eating is a progressive disease that wants me dead.

I didn't want to die, but I didn't want to admit to anyone I had "fallen off the wagon" either. As the calendar sped toward the holidays, I faced an endless progression of potlucks and parties. I thought my glory days were over; I thought any morning I would wake up fat again.

I was 170 pounds the day I scheduled the first operation. Twenty-four days later I was 197. I had gained 27 pounds in less than a month. I was binge-eating from 7,000 to 10,000 or more calories a day, so mathematically it *was* possible to gain that much that fast. But what was I thinking? Or rather, why *wasn't* I thinking?

Deep into the holiday season, I felt broken and defeated and completely joyless. One morning while listening to the radio on the way to work I realized my current theme song could very well be "Rudolph the Relapse Reindeer." It made me incredibly sad, but even that sobering thought didn't slow me down.

I couldn't stop the compulsive nature of this disease. Even then, as I was stuffing my second Egg McMuffin into my mouth, I was maneuvering my car from the golden arches straight to the espresso stand. Even then, I ordered a double mocha latte grande with extra whip cream and a package of chocolate covered espresso beans.

But when Christmas Eve arrived, I found the courage to light a candle during the evening church service and get down on my knees to pray for just one more miracle.

Kicking and screaming all the way to goal

Miracles *DO* happen.

In the depths of despair, when the light at the end of tunnel was certain to be an oncoming train, I turned back to what had worked before. I knew what I had to do; I knew I had to halt the progression of self will run riot.

I had to be willing to go to any length to enjoy the recovery I'd briefly tasted. There was a proven, workable solution to my problem, and for two and a half years I had walked this walk. It was time to find the strength within me to devote the rest of my life to staying on this path.

On Christmas Eve, the answer was as simple and as difficult as getting on my knees and asking for help. "God, grant me the serenity to accept the things I cannot change, the courage to change the things I can, and the wisdom to know the difference."

That one simple prayer was the answer. That one simple prayer helped me to turn the battleship, which had been moving full steam ahead toward cascading falls and certain destruction, with only an oar. I had forgotten that by asking God to direct the underwater currents and the force of the wind, one can, indeed, turn the ship around.

I had spent a month in physical and mental distress. I

had experienced constant indigestion and took TUMS by the handful. I was sneak eating, binge eating, and overeating by any name you want to call it. I blamed the full moon. I blamed PMS. I blamed the breakup with my gentleman friend. I had hot flashes, night sweats, hemorrhoids and anxiety attacks on a regular basis.

I had to relearn the phrase "Let go and let God." I had to believe God could relieve me, on a daily basis, of my compulsion to overeat. I had to surrender all my willfulness and trust in a power greater than myself.

I had to relearn humility. The hardest thing of all was finding the willingness to pick up the telephone and reconnect with those on this planet who had been holding my hand along the way.

At last, I finally called New York David, and admitted to him my program had been less than stellar during the previous month. I was afraid he would give up on me, but once again, I underestimated him.

"Honey," said NY David in the most angelic voice I'd ever heard, "taking the weight back is not an option. You're going to follow through, get to goal and have the excess skin removed. I know it. I've always known it. You're a winner, Honey. I'll always be here for you."

A sense of unimaginable calm descended over me. Yes, I thought, I am a winner. I am a miracle. God doesn't make junk. God wants the best for me. I owe it to God to be the best I can possibly be.

I returned my attention to what worked. I attended every support group meeting available, whether it dealt with food or other compulsive addictions. I re-read a pile of self-help literature. I renewed my commitment to my original food plan, including eating Subway low-fat sandwiches on a regular basis. I got my butt back to the gym. I walked on the beach or boardwalk every day when there wasn't a typhoon blowing.

And within another month and a half, I attained my personal goal. The numbers on the scale settled safely inside the 160s and I made a conscious effort not to lose any more weight. It was good enough; *I* was good enough.

"Cosmetic" surgery

After school one day in mid-February I plopped down in the chair facing the principal's desk. "If I decide to go through with this surgery, I'll be taking two weeks off. The one before and the one after spring break." I sighed. "I can still cancel, if you think that's too much time away from my classroom." I paused, and gazed out his window while he patiently waited for me to continue. I sighed again. "So what do you think I should do?"

My principal absentmindedly tapped his index finger on the small paperback book ever-present on his desk. I'd sought his counsel often enough to know the title of the book by heart: "Don't Sweat the Small Stuff…and it's all small stuff."

"But it's not small stuff," I argued, before he'd said a single word. "It's five procedures in two installments. I'd have to go under general anesthesia two times in the next four months, and full recovery would take me right up to the start of the next school year."

He smiled. "Do you want me to talk you out of it?"

"No." I shook my head. "Just tell me if it's the right thing to do."

"I can't tell you that," he said with a small shrug.

"Well, then what would *you* do?"

He laughed. And once I got over trying to look indignant, I laughed too. The thought of my favorite highly-energetic, not-an-ounce-of-fat-on-him, elementary principal needing to have excess skin removed after losing over 230 pounds was totally absurd.

"Okay." I took a deep breath, and checked the points off on my fingers as I spoke. "I've got enough sick leave. I've got two-thirds of the money in my savings account. I can borrow the rest against my annuities at just three percent interest. Six months from now I'll be completely healed. Two years from now I'll have the loan paid off and be putting money back into my savings account."

"So," said my principal, "you've decided to go ahead with it."

"Those were the pros," I replied. "I have yet to check off the cons."

"Cons?" He furrowed his brow. "What cons?"

"Well, like the fact that I'll have to miss two weeks of work."

"You said you've got enough sick time accrued."

I shrugged. "But what will people think about me using my sick leave for something other than actually being sick?" I looked him in the eye and held his gaze. "You know I value your opinion. Don't hold back. What do you think about this?"

He drew in a lungful of air and slowly expelled it. "I think you've just run quite the marathon," he said. "So why would you stop before stepping across the finish line?"

So in March, at what I considered a very healthy weight of 168, I plunked down $25,000 for a total of five skin-removal procedures over the course of two clinic inpatient sessions. Insurance deemed the whole thing "cosmetic," and would not pay a dime.

In for a penny, in for a pound, I ruefully told myself.

The first procedure involved three body areas, removing flab from my abdomen, upper thighs, and the "bat wings" removed from my upper arms.

Much more than a simple "tummy tuck," I had a complete circumferential abdominoplasty—the scar started on both sides of my spine, came clear around my belly, and I looked to all the world like I'd been cut totally in half, then sewn back together.

The scar was not straight, but angled up on one side, as they had tried to incorporate a previous jagged scar I'd gotten when I fell off a pair of metal stilts at age 13. "We tried to minimize the scar tissue on your stomach," my doctor said, but we had not previously discussed this, and I thought I looked like a drunken surgeon-in-training had tried to stitch me back up.

I was shocked when they sent me home after just two nights in a recovery unit. I still had three clear plastic "tennis balls" hanging by surgical tubing from inside the front incision. They were there to drain off the fluid that might pool under what was left of the skin. I had to unscrew the collection balls every morning, and pour the pinkish fluid into a measuring cup. Then I called the doctor's office as soon as they opened to report the total amount and color of the fluid.

"You're doing fine," they reassured me. "You're right on schedule."

The swelling across my belly was horrific, but I could see a vast improvement in the way I looked the very first day. They had reinserted my navel and stitched it in at the appropriate spot. I had told them not to bother, but was told it was a "point of reference," and they had to do it anyway. I wondered how much that little extra had cost me.

The balls and tubing were removed after 10 days, but I took an additional week of sick leave before I felt recovered enough to return to work. Even then, I developed an abscess in one of the abdominal drainage sites. An ultrasound confirmed it was nothing more than fluid, and it was aspirated without further complication.

The first of July I went back to have my butt lifted, and my breasts put back up where they belonged. For days before the procedures, I had nightmares about either my breasts being way too high and tucked under my chin, or about one of them being placed significantly higher than the other one.

It is odd that I did not worry about my nipple size being reduced by more than half, because that is exactly what happened. I ended up with almost no areolas, not much more than buds, really, and I lost a lot of sensitivity. None of this was fully explained before my surgery, and I felt undeniably ugly and mutilated. I deeply grieved this change in my sexuality, and fell into a long period of post-surgical depression.

And speaking of sexuality—I'd now have the embarrassing task of explaining the mishmash of prominent scars all over my body to any future potential lovers. From my elbows to armpit, from the nipples down to a line clear across my chest, all across my abdomen, wrapping back to my spine, and from my inner thighs back up under my buttocks, I was a poorly-drawn road map.

Some skin still sagged and the wrinkles were virtually everywhere. My body was not perfect; I was not 20 years old. My body was covered with the glorious battle scars of a war that is waged daily by every compulsive overeater on the entire planet.

But the overhanging bulk of flabby skin, the 8 to 10 inch

abomination they referred to as "an apron" was gone, and for that, I gave thanks.

No secrets in a small town

The middle-aged woman waiting in the grocery checkout line ahead of me, an acquaintance whose name I couldn't even recall, turned to me and quite abruptly inquired, "So how much weight have you lost?"

My first reaction was to tell her to mind her own damned business. What nerve!

But almost instantaneously, my second reaction was the internal acknowledgment it might behoove me to just relax and enjoy the attention of my recent physical transformation—a transformation for which I was deeply awed and grateful.

"I've lost more than you weigh," I said quietly.

"No way!" she exclaimed, her eyes widening. "Not possible!" Then she lowered her voice to a slightly confessional tone and leaned uncomfortably close. "I'm a little over 200 pounds," she admitted. "Well, actually, I haven't stepped on a scale in some time. I'm probably somewhere close to 230."

I couldn't help it. I grinned like a Cheshire cat. "Like I said, I've lost more than you weigh."

She shook her head in disbelief. "Good for you." She whispered again. "Good. For. You."

Living at Goal Weight

My "weight window" fluctuated between 165 and 175 for over three years—from early in 2002 to late in 2005. Every time the numbers on the scale approached the top end of what qualified as "acceptable," I took up the slack and worked my program a little harder.

In the fall of 2002, I wrote an inspirational weight-recovery story, submitted it to Guidepost Magazine, and they almost instantly called me! They wanted it for their March, 2003, publication!

They sent a professional photographer from Longview to come photograph me happily walking the boardwalk along the beach. The wind blew my hair sideways that day, but nothing could erase my beaming smile.

Also in the fall of 2002, at my 30-year class reunion, I shared my weight-loss journey with a select few of my former classmates. One of them, obviously touched by my story, immediately offered me a quantity of his "frequent flyer miles" so I could go to New York to meet my mentor David. I accepted, and during spring break of 2003, exactly a year after my skin removal surgery, I flew to Manhattan and met my Angel/Eskimo/Cheerleader face-to-face.

New York David and I spent a week seeing the sights of the city that never sleeps, and I had a fabulous time. He was exactly the same in person as he'd been on the phone, and we laughed and talked like we'd been friends forever.

I'd left home with 35 things I wanted to see and do on my trip, and we managed to cross 31 of them off the list in 7 short days. It was a dream come true to be able to keep up with him when we walked all over the lower part of the island. I even convinced him to walk with me across Brooklyn Bridge, so I could boast having traversed major bridges on both coasts!

We went up in the Empire State Building, rode in a handsome cab around Central Park, took the boat to see the Statue of Liberty, and yes, I really did wear the red sequined dress to go out for a night on the town!

While in Manhattan, I also got to meet the Guidepost editor who'd worked with me on my story. I toured the offices, met a lot of high-power people, and was treated like a celebrity. She even took David and me to lunch at a nearby French bistro. All three of us ordered a healthy meal, but since I'd been doing so much walking, I gave in and indulged a bit by splitting a decadent dessert with her.

I came home from my week in New York weighing just four pounds heavier, which I considered a minor miracle. I got right back into my regular routine, and it took me three concerted weeks to take those four pounds back off.

Weight maintenance was entirely new territory for me. My entire life I'd always been either gaining or losing. Maintaining consistency on the scale was a new trick I needed to learn. Often I felt like I was walking a tight rope. Eating well and exercising daily kept me balanced, but I often worried about falling back into the abyss.

I constantly counted on the help of my village, my friends, my support group, and most of all, my Higher Power. Together we'd been able to do what I could have never done alone. On October 10, 1999, I had found not only hope, but the willingness to surrender my compulsive eating to a power greater than myself.

After three years of successful maintenance, which included completing the annual 6.2 mile Astoria/Meglar Bridge Walk two more times (*improving my time with each crossing*), I thought I truly had it made.

CHAPTER VIII: RELAPSE?! Are you freakin' kidding me?

The Elephant Man and me

In the 1980 film "The Elephant Man," all John Merrick wanted to do was be like everybody else. He wanted to be able to lie down and sleep in a normal bed like a normal person. But he was not a normal person, never would be, and his refusal to accept life on life's terms ultimately led to his undoing, and his death.

I, too, just wanted to be normal. I wanted to fit in. I wanted to be like everybody else. I desperately wanted to be able to "eat like a normal person." But I'm not a normal person, and I never will be. I am a compulsive overeater.

Complacency is the enemy. Complacency is a killer. Complacency tricked me into thinking I could relax my food limitations "just this once."

But it's the first compulsive bite that gets us fat, and eternal vigilance is required. We cannot rest on our laurels. I knew this clear down to my toes, and yet I apparently had to test the theory one more time.

I stopped regularly attending my support group. I thought I didn't need to stay connected to others who waged the same war. I thought maybe I could have just one bite of a maple bar, or just one handful of M&M peanuts. I thought I could handle buffet lines and potlucks.

Hadn't I suffered enough? Hadn't I paid my dues? Wasn't it time to be rid of the public stigma of always having to abstain from eating like others did?

I'd like to say unequivocally the compulsion to overeat was removed on a daily basis, but the truth was that some days the compulsion was removed, and some days it wasn't. The lines blurred further when I stopped keeping a daily food journal. I thought I didn't need to write down what I ate every day—I was at goal weight now! I was normal!

And I was treading a very slippery slope.

Rationally, I knew that even smelling maple bars was likely to push me over the edge, and M&M peanuts were nothing more than little chocolate-covered hand grenades. Yet I couldn't stop myself from pushing the limits of continued recovery.

One big, fat, fraud

I had 25,000 reasons to maintain my goal weight, and each one of them had a dollar tag attached to it. I'd gone through hell and high water to be able to wear size 8 jeans, and blouses with a simple "L" on the tag, or maybe even an occasional "M." Why in the world would I not move heaven and earth to keep the numbers on the scale right there where they belonged?

But it turned out moving heaven and earth was a piece of cake (*pun intended*) compared to the challenge of resisting the daily temptation of compulsive overeating. I fought tooth and nail, but the numbers kept creeping up.

I equated the struggle to hold my weight down to trying to hold dozens of ping-pong balls under water. The more I tried to hold them down, the more they struggled to rise to the surface. Eventually, the pressure I put on them was so great, and it built up so much resistance, when they popped free, they zinged way up into the atmosphere.

For over three full years I stayed inside the target zone, and all the while my disease had been busy doing push-ups in the corner, biding its time, waiting for me to totally succumb to the killer of complacency.

About the time I rebounded past the 200-pound mark, people I hardly knew stopped me on the street—or in the grocery store—to ask me what had happened. Others simply looked at me with sad eyes, then looked away and shook their heads in disgust.

So what the hell *had* happened?

Figuring there had to be something wrong with the way my brain processed things, I returned to counseling for psychological answers. But the woman who'd kicked me in the butt back in 1999 was no longer practicing in the area, and I had to seek out another counselor. She listened, she nodded, but she wasn't cut from the same cloth as the firecracker who'd grabbed me by the shirtfront and barked concrete directions in my face.

Nevertheless, my time in the counselor's office gave me much to think about during the two weeks in between. So I thought, and I ate, and I thought some more. I wasn't taking the whole thing too seriously, but at least I could tell those who pried I was "seeing a counselor" in hushed tones, which immediately shut them up.

Slowly, as my weight continued to rise, and with the counselor's gentle guidance, I began to formulate some theories about what was going on inside me.

I had retired from teaching in June, 2006, a part of me had became terribly disoriented, and I had imploded. I'd been a teacher for 30 years—it defined me. So since I no longer taught, who was I?

The quest to redefine myself was arduous, and in my haste to make an instant transition, I made a lot of mistakes. Although I made a business plan, and thought I knew exactly where I was going, it turned out to be a poor decision. I spent thousands of dollars on a website, brochures, and business cards, but my goals were not clearly defined.

I had created what I called an "Umbrella Company," and it covered the various "occupations" I thought I could successfully juggle: Life Coach, Writer, Editor, Workshop Presenter, Public Speaker, and so forth.

With the focus so blurry, I became a jack of all trades, and master of none. The business never had a chance to get off the ground, and I felt humiliated and shamed. If anyone asked me a simple "what do you do?" question, I turned red with embarrassment.

Naturally, I coped with the stress by eating.

During this time, I entered into relationship after relationship, each lasting about five months. It got to be a joke among my friends. "Why is five months the magic number?" they asked. And the only answer I could manage was a rueful, "That's when the tops of their heads open up and the snakes crawl out."

In hindsight, these quasi-relationships were simply rescue missions. I thought I could help these men realize their potentials. Falling in love with a guy's potential became a specialty of mine, and I can honestly say that I left each one better than when I'd found him.

"Haven't you ever dated *up*?" a friend asked.

"Up?"

"Have you ever dated a guy with more education, more money, or more ambition than you?" She raised one eyebrow and continued, "Have you ever even dated a guy who was your true equal?"

I ate over that little insight, too, trying to stuff down the uncomfortable truth.

My life coaching studies had taught me there are five major areas in which we all must find balance and harmony: career, finances, relationships, health and fitness, and spirituality.

All five of these categories were my own personal disaster areas. I had no real career any more, my savings were being rapidly depleted, despite having recently been a "normal" weight, I couldn't find a satisfactory relationship, my health and fitness goals were now totally in the toilet and my spirituality was completely non-existent, as I felt my Higher Power had abandoned me.

Despite my best intentions, I had fallen headfirst into the abyss I had so desperately hoped to avoid. The pain and humiliation of relapse became the ultimate Catch-22: I gained weight because I overate, and I overate because I had gained weight.

I was one big, fat, fraud.

Once more, with enthusiasm!

Son-of-a-gun, I had rested on my laurels, and, *what a surprise!* my laurels had gotten bigger. I had to buy larger clothes, I shunned looking into mirrors, and I didn't want to be seen in public. I isolated—and overeating is a disease of isolation. I tried not to care. I tried to shrug it off, pretend it couldn't be helped, and blame what I called my insurmountable fat genetic set point.

Trying to joke my way around my obvious distress, I

told people "some of us have to be fat so that the rest of you will look good." Self-deprecating humor had never served me, but I couldn't stop. My picture could have been placed in the dictionary next to the word miserable. I was the classic poster child of despair.

But how does one go about reclaiming emotional and physical sanity? Where does one start? Where is the switch that must be flipped? Is it possible to come back from such a devastating relapse? How could I turn the battleship around, *yet again,* with only that one single oar?

The mental image of that last question intrigued me, and I stopped my pity party in its tracks to contemplate the question: How can a battleship be turned around when I have only one puny little oar? Somewhere in the recesses of my memory, I was sure I had once known the answer to this conundrum. Was the answer still in there?

Out on the Columbia River, ocean-going ships often anchor in close to Tongue Point to wait for the tide to change. On a flood tide, it's much easier for an outgoing vessel to cross the bar, or a Portland-bound ship to travel upstream. Therefore, it's only prudent for them to capitalize on nature's help.

Nature's help. Hhmm... If one had the tide, the wind, and the river current all working in your favor, then one could reasonably argue you actually could turn the battleship with an oar... right?

Tentatively inspired, I went looking for my bootstraps.

The Law of Attraction

I can honestly say I did not find my bootstraps—my bootstraps found me!

The very next day after I said, "Well, okay, maybe I can do this," I was invited to a four-session workshop held in Astoria. I accepted, as I could find no excuse not to, and commuted with a couple other gals once a week to learn about "The Law of Attraction."

At the very first class, something resonated within me with such force it took my breath away. I immediately ordered the book being used, and read it cover-to-cover before the next class. It was "The Law of Attraction: The Science of Getting More of What You Want, and Less of What You Don't," by Michael Losier.

What you put your energy, attention, and focus on grows larger, wrote Michael. The Universe resonates with our vibrations. We attract more of whatever we bring into our vibrational bubble. However, he cautioned, the Universe does not hear us when we say "Don't, No, and Not," so you must choose your words carefully.

I had to think on that awhile, but it suddenly dawned on me. I'd been saying "I don't want to gain my weight back," and the Universe only heard my energy, attention, and focus was on *GAINING MY WEIGHT BACK*.

Change your thinking, and change your life, wrote Michael. Thoughts are powerful. Thoughts become words, words become reality.

Over the course of the next few months, I regularly gathered a dozen "like-minded" others around my dining room table and together we actively practiced The Law of Attraction. The results were nothing short of flabbergasting. Every single one of us attracted some form of what we sought, be it a new job, new relationship, more money, or greater fitness.

"Michael Losier lives in Victoria," I told the group one day, holding up his book. "I don't know when, or how, but I'm destined to meet him."

The Universe heard me, and immediately responded. I met Michael for the first time less than a month later, in Calgary, Alberta. I asked if I could take his photo to show my friends "back home," and he turned me down.

"No pictures," he said, his eyes twinkling, "unless you're in them with me." He took my camera and handed it to his assistant. Then he put his arm around me and told me to "Say cheese."

In the context of his book, I had neglected to ask for what I really wanted, or give the Universe permission to bring me "this, or something more." Thankfully, Michael is one terrific guru, and the picture with him became one of my greatest inspirational treasures.

Returning home, I began to objectively approach my problems as if I were my own life-coaching client.

In the area of career, I decided to official close my catch-all business and concentrate on what I felt best suited me—writing. And if some editing clients happened to come my way, they would be most welcome.

As for finances, I examined my teaching pension and created a workable budget, which included putting a little into my savings account each month.

Then I ever-so-gently detached myself from a man whom I loved, but who wasn't the right man for me for the long-term. It was bittersweet, but necessary, and his family will always be very dear to me.

Spiritually, I began regularly attending support groups again, and surrounded myself with more like-minded people. Whether called Divine Spirit, Universal Mind, Higher Power, or God, there was something out there— some Energy Source, to which I needed to sit up and pay more attention.

All that was left to tackle was the elephant on the table—again! My health and fitness begged for my attention, energy, and focus, and I returned that area to top spot on my list of self-improvement priorities.

Pedaling my ass off

My knee doctor suggested three low-impact activities to build my thigh strength while losing weight: swimming, recumbent biking, and walking. He preferred swimming and biking, as walking was technically weight-bearing, and as he unnecessarily pointed out, my knees were not going to be able to carry this much weight forever.

"Every pound on your body," he told me, "puts four pounds of pressure on your knees."

I did the math. "So you're saying losing 20 pounds relieves 80 pounds of pressure?"

He tilted his head and frowned. "Twenty pounds won't be enough to get the relief you seek. You're going to need to lose a lot more than that—probably closer to 100 pounds would be ideal."

I didn't say anything. His estimation was dead-on. I accepted the paper he handed me listing his prioritized exercise recommendations, got corticosteroid injections in both knees, and got the heck out of his office, my cheeks flaming red with embarrassment.

But I'd heard him, and somewhere inside me I found the wherewithal to swallow my pride and take affirmative action. Once again, it was about becoming willing.

And it was that willingness that led me to check the Fred Meyer sale ads the following week. Sure enough, heavy-duty recumbent bikes were on sale. By combining the sale price with an extra 15% off coupon in the newspaper ad, and I could get a pretty decent bike.

I found a friend to put the bike together for me, got a large piece of plywood to protect the carpet in my rec room, and placed the bike facing the television set.

"How long before it becomes just another expensive clothes rack?" asked the very first friend who saw the bike.

I'm not sure I'd recommend this type of inspiration for others, but speaking only for myself, getting pissed off is a very strong motivator.

"On the phone, on the bike" became my new mantra. Now I won't say I spend too much time yakking, but the hours/miles/calories started adding up right away. The temptation was to tell myself "You've burned 50 calories, so you can have an Oreo cookie and it won't count," but I managed to resist that temptation by staying pissed off at the naysayers.

In my food journal, I began recording my exercise each day. Even if all I did was a few simple stretches, I wrote it down. When I rode the bike, I wrote the time, the miles pedaled, and the approximate calories expended.

Then I added one more dimension: If I wanted to sit in front of the TV in the rec room, I had to get on the bike.

Within the first month, friends started noticing my weight loss, and I knew the pedaling was paying off in tangible results.

In the land of Oz

One of the shows I began saving daily on DVR was the Dr. Oz show. Since it aired in the middle of the afternoon, I'd rarely seen it, but I'd seen Dr. Oz on Oprah, and had been impressed. His teaching style and my learning style were pretty much in sync, and I suspected there was much I could learn about health and fitness from him.

Using the DVR, it was easy to catch up every morning while I was on the bike, and I could fast-forward all those pesky commercials, too! Right away, I learned to keep a notebook handy, as I needed to jot down things to investigate in greater detail later.

"So if Dr. Oz says it, it must be true?" teased a friend of mine I met for lunch a few weeks later.

My face flushed. "Sorry if you think I'm worshipping at his feet," I replied. "It's just that I know he's got a whole team of experts to draw from, so there's a better than average chance it's always pretty darn good information."

She shook her head. "Well, whatever you're doing, it seems to be working."

"That's just it," I replied. "There's no one way to get where your body needs to go. No one right way to lose weight. Dr. Oz offers suggestions, and I follow through on the ones that happen to grab me at the moment." I shrugged. "Nobody could, or should, do it all."

"Oh yeah?" she challenged. "Name one thing you've not done that Dr. Oz said was good for you."

"I don't eat almonds."

My friend laughed. "You're allergic to almonds," she replied, rolling her eyes.

"You said name one thing," I countered. Then I ordered my turkey sandwich on wheat, no mayo, no cheese, lots of veggies, and a squiggle of mustard.

"So Dr. Oz doesn't like mayo or cheese?" She raised an accusatory eyebrow.

"Dr. Oz has pointed out the amount of unnecessary fat we unconsciously consume each day. I don't need mayo or cheese to enjoy my sandwich."

She narrowed her eyes, and I believe out of spite, ordered a meatball sub with double cheese, and no veggies at all. "Suit yourself, but I'm not going to be deprived."

I didn't answer her. I was beginning to look upon food as merely fuel, and I was simply choosing the fuel with the highest octane and lowest emissions and carbon footprint, so to speak. I never felt deprived—feeling deprived would drive me to overeat, sure as anything. I simply chose to honor my body, and get the most nutrition out of the calories I put in.

Daily, I either learned something new, or something I already knew was reinforced, or perhaps fine-tuned.

After watching one Dr. Oz show, I knew I needed more fiber in my diet. Dr. Oz is big on poop—the color and shape and consistency—and I decided to experiment with natural ways to increase my daily fiber.

I bought in bulk, then put together dozens of afternoon "snack packs" consisting of two prunes, three dates, and a half dozen walnut halves. Within two weeks, I noticed my midday energy had increased, and my poop was more regular. Plus, I got an extra benefit from the Omega 3s in the walnuts.

My knee doc had been the one to suggest bumping up my Omega 3s by taking fish oil supplements. But after watching a Dr. Oz show on Omega 3s, I switched my fish oil to krill oil.

"I have a present for you," said my friend at lunch the

next month. She dug into her oversized purse and handed me a pair of purple latex gloves. "You can pretend you're The Assistant of the Day."

"You've been watching Dr. Oz!"

"I've been watching your transformation the past few months, and I thought it couldn't hurt to tune in now and then." She scowled. "But there's no way anybody would ever get me into that Truth Tube of his!"

I nodded, but I knew I'd already stepped into a Truth Tube of my own. I had become fully aware of not only the honest numbers on the scale, but also my blood pressure, resting heart rate, fasting blood sugar, HDL and LDL cholesterol, waist measurement, and BMI. And I knew which exercises, foods, and supplements would help me get to my optimum, but realistic, goals.

Dr. Oz told me to stretch like a cat every morning—and I did. He told me to move 30 minutes a day—and I did that, too. He said not to eat within three hours of bedtime—and I didn't. He said all snacks had to be smaller than the size of your fist—and I began snacking on the individual bags of microwave popcorn, not cheating by ingesting the larger one filled with 2½ servings.

Pistachios were addicting. After several attempts to stop with the recommended portion, I had to admit defeat and cut them out completely.

Dr. Oz said that smart dieting was a marathon, not a sprint—and I wholeheartedly embraced that notion.

Dr. Oz said his goal was to make America healthier, and to help him do that, he asked we tell just one other person about something we'd learned. Always an overachiever, I did far better than that—I started telling anyone and everyone exactly how I was accomplishing my complete health transformation.

I also proclaimed that someday, in the not-to-distant future, I'd be on the Dr. Oz show. I told them I was "riding my recumbent bike to New York" at the rate of about 15 miles per day. I assured friends that 3,000 miles was nothing compared to my determination, and I'd soon be there, pulling on the purple gloves and holding up a quantity of belly fat, helping Dr. Oz spread the word about the dangerous complications of obesity.

Of course, my friends raised a few eyebrows, but they only told me to let them know when to tune in—no one dared argue with the kind of positive changes they were seeing in me.

And then one day, Dr. Oz introduced me to something totally new—a concept uncomfortably contrary to all my previously-held weight-loss beliefs. He encouraged me to add an additional "supplement" to his previous OTC suggestions to bolster optimum weight loss.

My all-time favorite fruit

My initial weight loss, from 1999 through 2002, had been without the use of any particular diet aids. I had been adamant about the fact that I had released 231 pounds without bypass surgery, exercising to the point of obsession, or popping any pills.

Although often tempted by "the quick fix," I had never resorted to taking anything purported to be an "appetite suppressant," or "fat blaster." I lumped those claims into the miracle snake oil category, and stuck with the tried and true—calories taken in must be less than calories being burned to see the numbers on the scale go down.

Then one day I saw Dr. Oz do a demonstration on the

effect of taking raspberry ketone supplements. He held up two little red inflated balloons and suggested they were fat cells. When he donned safety glasses and surrounded the balloons with liquid nitrogen, the balloons dramatically decreased in size.

"Raspberry ketones temporarily shrink your fat cells," he said. "They trick your body into thinking you're already thin."

"They break up the fat cells and help your body burn fat," said his guest that day, weight-loss expert Lisa Lynn.

I've always been a visual learner, and his graphic demonstration struck such a strong chord with me that I decided it couldn't hurt to do a little more research.

I read that raspberry ketone is the primary aroma compound of red raspberries. The compound helps control adiponectin, a protein used by the body to regulate metabolism.

My mind flashed back to 1979. Vividly, I remembered my local physician, a man I greatly admired, asking me if I'd like to do an experiment with him. He told me exactly what to eat for dinner that night, to weigh and measure the portions, and to complete my meal by 6 p.m.

I did as told, and was waiting in the parking lot when his office opened the next morning. He gave me syrup of ipecac, and I immediately vomited. There, in my vomit, one could clearly make out the various components of my dinner, finished 15 hours before.

"I figured as much," he said thoughtfully.

"Shouldn't I have digested all that by now?" I asked.

"Your metabolism is..." He paused, searching for the right words. "Very efficient. You extract every single calorie from your food." He patted my shoulder. "You'll be the last to go in a famine."

There was no consolation in his words; my metabolism had flat-lined.

So now I wondered if these raspberry ketones might give my metabolism the jumpstart it had always desired. I was almost embarrassed to admit I was grasping at straws—looking for "the softer easier way" to lose weight.

But Dr. Oz had said it was the "Number one miracle in a bottle to burn your fat." And if Dr. Oz said it was worth a try, I was willing.

Research said there were no side effects, and there was no caffeine. It would be like eating 90 pounds of raspberries twice a day, but without the calories. Raspberries had always been my favorite fruit, so I took that as a sign.

Naturally, my Internet exploration revealed a catch: One must take the supplement paired with regular exercise and a well-balanced diet of healthy whole foods for optimum benefits.

No problem! I was already exercising and eating well, so maybe these ketones were the ticket to start eating, and living, like an already-thin person.

Maybe all I needed to see the desired results was a booster shot of a natural hormone—adiponectin. I ordered some online that very day.

Staying the course—against all odds

Lisa Lynn, the weight-loss expert Dr. Oz had consulted, said the longer a person stays on the raspberry ketones, the bigger the results. She said most people were likely see some change after five days.

Dr. Oz had shown pictures of women who'd taken the supplement, and the changes were dramatic. He said that some women didn't ever want to come off them.

I could relate. Taking raspberry ketones a half hour before lunch and dinner became one of the only things I could "control" in 2013. I wasn't sure it was helping, but I wasn't about to take the chance I'd spiral out of orbit if I stopped taking them.

The bottom line with most supplements, and even with some prescribed medications, is if you believe it will work, it probably will. It's the placebo effect. The mind tells you that taking a pill will make you better, and the body follows through with the desired result.

In March, 2013, both my favorite aunt and my mother passed away. Twelve days apart, and buried side-by-side, the matriarchs of our family rested in peace—but there was no peace for those remaining. Our dysfunctional family dynamics escalated to an excruciating level.

Oh how I wanted to self-medicate with food! I wanted to fall face-down into any and all high-calorie, sugary, salty, non-nutritional substances I could find. I just wanted to "comfort" myself by stuffing copious amounts of food into my mouth. Any kind of food would do! Just gimme!

But an odd thing happened. By now, taking raspberry ketones twice a day had become a deeply ingrained habit. And I discovered first-hand how hard it is to break a habit—even a good one! So I kept taking my supplements, kept walking, or swimming, or riding my recumbent bike, and kept telling myself that "food won't fix it."

The next month a former boyfriend took his own life. The month after that, his father, a man who'd been like a father to me, died of a heart attack. His wife immediately moved closer to her own family, and I felt the sharp pain of additional abandonment. Then my travelling companion of many years had to be hospitalized for a month due to heart problems and we had to cancel a European cruise—a trip we'd eagerly anticipated for a full year.

Still, I clung to the routine of taking my raspberry ketones. On Facebook, my friends often saw me write the words that had become my constant mantra: Stay the Course! Stay the Course! Whatever the hell else happens, just Stay. The. Course!

And most amazingly, my body rewarded me for my efforts and returned to a height/weight proportionate number before the end of the year.

But the goal line had moved!

Previously, as in a mere decade ago, 168 pounds looked darn good on my body. Back then, I'd worn size 8 slacks to work, and they had fastened comfortably around my waist even before I had all the skin removed.

But now, those same slacks were too tight for me to button. Apparently, during my "decade of indifference," my body had shape-shifted! Call it the inevitable middle-age spread if you want, but the hands of time had slapped me squarely across the face. The pain was almost unbearable. *Why wasn't it still enough?!*

After what I considered a reasonable period of denial and mourning, like about two weeks, I decided it was time to reevaluate my self-proclaimed "goal." If 168 wasn't "good enough," then what number would be? I arbitrarily decided another 15 pounds down might do it.

At 153, I could finally button those pants without cutting myself in two. I set my "maintenance window" at 150-155, but I kept taking the ketones, afraid to let go of my metabolic security blanket.

Meanwhile, Dr. Oz had abandoned the practice of broadcasting a person's weight when they stepped into the Truth Tube. Instead, he suggested judging your overall health not by the number on the scale, by your waist measurement.

"Your waist measurement should be less than half your height," said Dr. Oz.

Although I'd always been 5'6", or 66", my doctor had recently recorded my height at 5-foot 5, or 65 inches. Shrinking my height naturally impacted my goal waist measurement.

According to Dr. Oz's calculations, my waistline should be less than 32 and one-half inches. But at 153 pounds, my actual waist measurement was right around 34.5 inches.

I started doing crunches with a vengeance, hoping to spot-reduce my waist. I added some weight lifting as well— nothing too strenuous, just working to tone the muscles of my upper body, hoping the muscle would encourage my body to burn the fat of my belly.

When Dr. Oz did a segment on omentum, I felt my spirit implode. The greater omentum is the apron-like fold of visceral peritoneum (*membrane*) that hangs down from the stomach and extends from the greater curvature beneath the ribs down in front of the small intestines. The fat stored there is often responsible for coronary artery disease, high cholesterol, and diabetes.

I was devastated; after all my hard work, was I still at a higher health risk for these maladies?

Grasping at straws, I considered having the fat sucked out through liposuction. It was costly, it was risky, and I might end with unsatisfactory final results.

I took a step back and reviewed the overall picture. My WC (*waist circumference*) was 34.5. My BMI (*body mass index*) was 25, which teetered right on the line between normal and overweight. But then I stumbled across a brand-spanking-new health indicator on the horizon. In the April, 2014 edition of "O Magazine," I read about ABSI (*a body shape index*), which takes into account weight, height, and waist circumference.

I quickly looked up the online ABSI calculator. *AH-HA!* According to their calculations, I was at a below-average risk for dying from any obesity-related maladies.

So instead of spending my savings on a liposuction procedure that carried no guarantee I'd be any healthier as a result of undergoing such a treatment, I decided to spend the money on a new car—a Mustang!

My weight leveled off between 143 and 145 (*the actual number on my driver's license!*) and in June, 2014, I turned 60. Back when I weighed 396, I bought a car simply because I could fit into it. Back then, I'd placed another Mustang on my list of ultimate weight-loss goals. And now, I have one—Kona blue with sparkling blue racing stripes!

Phooey and pshaw on those who think my waist should be any smaller. I was/am healthy, and happy, and I'm much more than just "good enough"—I'm fabulous!

One day at a time

There is no cure for compulsive overeating. One must surrender to the disease on a daily basis and embrace what works. The research has proven, beyond any doubt, that keeping a daily food journal is key to not only losing weight, but in maintaining one's goal weight.

My preferred food journal is a compact 4 x 5 ½ inches spiral bound. It tucks right into my purse or in the top compartment of my suitcase, or in the jockey box in my car. In other words, I keep it handy!

Each day I record the date, my morning weight, and the food that goes into my mouth throughout the day, along with the approximate portion size and calories. My target calories are somewhere between 1200 and 1500, but naturally, there are exceptions.

In addition, I write down "Yes!" after "Meds?" when I've taken my seven daily over-the-counter supplements: a multi-vitamin, calcium (*with extra vitamin D*), CoQ10, krill oil, resveratol, glucosamine, and Sam-e. And finally, I log in the amount of exercise I've gotten that day—the type, time, and if known, the number of calories burned.

I ride my recumbent bike for 30 to 90 minutes almost every day. On days when I don't ride the bike, I often get in a walk or a trip to the pool. Movement is essential, and I rarely have days when I record nothing under exercise.

On a daily basis, I am grateful to be relieved of the compulsion to overeat. But I'm not perfect. I still have occasional screw-ups. And when I do, I write it all down anyway! Then I forgive myself for being human and get right back with the program the very next day.

Eternal vigilance—At first it sounds like more than anyone can handle, but don't let it discourage you. You only have to do this for one day—just for today. And one day at a time, you can achieve that happy and healthy body you seek.

So when would *"NOW"* be a good time for you to join me in the quest for better health?

EPILOGUE:
So What's the Plan?

On March 18, 2014, the first segment on the Dr. Oz show was "Are you a food addict? Take the test to find out!"

I responded to the title question, even before answering affirmatively to all five questions, with a loud and heartfelt, "Well, Duh!" But I stuck around to listen to the three-step plan that the expert, who said she was a "former" food addict, suggested in order to break the cycle.

Her suggestions were a page taken straight from my support group meetings:

1) Create a stopgap to your eating. HALT: Are you Hungry, Angry, Lonely, or Tired? Set a timer for 10 minutes to stay away from the food while you decide.

2) Treat trigger foods as though they were alcohol to an alcoholic. Get them out of the house! The junk has to go! Get them out of your house, car, office desk drawer, etc.

3) Commit to not eating anything out of the bag, or out of the box, for two weeks. Detox your brain and your body.

And then, when my darling Dr. Oz said, "Once an alcoholic, always an alcoholic," I could have kissed him. To my way of thinking, based upon years of thorough personal and widespread research, there is no "cure" for the food addict. You can have recovery from your food addiction, one day at a time, but you must be forever vigilant.

That said, I have given a lot of thought to what I will do differently this time to prevent another relapse, and I've settled on my own three-point intervention:

1) I'm going public by publishing my story. Figuratively speaking, I'm not shoving my story of weight-loss recovery into the bottom drawer this time. Ten years ago, publishers passed it over, saying that since I wasn't a celebrity, no one would want to read my book. But today, through the magic of self-publishing, I'm getting the word out despite their apparent short-sightedness.

2) I've created a "Back from Obesity" Facebook page specifically dedicated to this book, and welcome readers to share in an open dialogue about issues with weight loss and maintenance. You're all now a part of my online health and fitness support group, and together we can do what we could never do alone.

3) I'm making myself available to work individually with others. Consider me your personal "Weight Loss Coach." It is through teaching one truly begins to understand, and by helping others achieve, and maintain, weight loss, I'm hoping to keep a handle on the numbers lighting up my scale, too. Send me a private message on the Facebook page and let's get started.

Thanks to everyone who read my story. I send you best wishes for health and happiness, always, and in all ways! If I can do it, you can do it too!

ABOUT THE AUTHOR

Long Beach, Washington, author Jan Bono has had five collections of humorous personal experience stories published, as well as two poetry chapbooks, one book of short romance, nine one-act plays, and a full-length dinner theater play. She's written for numerous magazines ranging from Guidepost to Star to Woman's World and has had 28 stories included in the Chicken Soup for the Soul series in the last five years. Jan was Grand Prize winner in the Coast Weekend serial mystery chapter-writing contest in 2012 and is currently writing a cozy mystery series set on the southwest Washington coast.

See more of Jan's work, and follow her blog: www.JanBonoBooks.com